COMBATING
ARTHRITIS

COMBATING
ARTHRITIS

Dr. RITU ARORA
B.H.M.S. (DLI) *(GOLD MEDALIST)*
M.D. (A.M.); DIP. ACUPUNCTURE
DIP. MAGNETOTHERAPY
DIP. N.D.D.Y.

B. JAIN PUBLISHERS (P) LTD
NEW DELHI

Note

Any information given in this book is not intended to be taken as a replacement for medical advice. Any person with a condition requiring medical attention should consult a qualified practitioner or therapist.

Reprint Edition: 2003
1st edition : 1999

Price: Rs. 110. 00

© Copyright with the Author

Published by :
Kuldeep Jain
For
B. Jain publishers (P.) Ltd.
1921, Street No. 10, Chuna Mandi,
Paharganj, New Delhi 110 055 (INDIA)
Phones: 2358 0800, 2358 1100, 2358 1300
Fax: 011-2358 0471

Printed in India by:
Unisons Techno Financial Consultants (P) Ltd.
522, FIE, Patpar Ganj, Delhi - 110 092

ISBN : 81-7021- 895-0
BOOK CODE : BR-5375

DEDICATED
TO MY PARENTS

INTRODUCTION

Arthritis owes it's origin to the very beginning of evolution which started changing it's forms with the advent and progress of human civilization. Several studies and researches have been carried out regarding the diagnosis, management and treatment but till date we have not been in a position to find even a single unique system which helps the patients.

It is basically the root of arthritis, its presentations that now more emphasis is being given to the alternative system of medicines rather only the orthodox system of medicine..

Oh! Doctor look I am suffering from arthritis. Kindly help me. "Take a pain killer and do the exercise "No" definitely "No" being a responsible social citizen of society, we as medical practitioners should always guide the patients regarding the illness, it's management, complications, possibility of cure and necessary precautions.

Arthritis is a crippling disease, which if not taken care can completely cripple human life.

Therefore it is the moral duty of each practitioner whether practising any system of medicine to make the society aware of the practical implications of arthritis. Keeping in mind all these practical aspects I have taken arthritis as the subject of presentation with all possible ways of helping a patient. At certain stage, we must truly recognize that at every step our aim is just not to cure but manage and treat also. We must study the subject with an open mind keeping in view the advantages and disadvantages of the available therapeutic kits.

I have tried my best to provide all possible details related to arthritis and rheumatology which includes diagnosis, treatment and management which is truly applicable for all of us specially to know the scope of each pathy. It not only enhances our knowledge but also makes us aware "About our scope" So that "The best guidance" is given to the patients.

I have given both the positive and negative results so that the scope is never under or over estimated. All the details of this work regarding clinical cases have been conducted at "We care health and Diagnostic centre". B-4/22 Paschim Vihar which has all the facilities including physiotherapy and acupuncture. It has been done under the able guidance of Dr. S.T. Wanjari Sr. Physiotherapist working in "Institution of physically handicaps".

I hope this small work will help each one of us to overcome big barriers, to understand this field and to guide our patients sincerely. It no where aims at criticizing any system but analyzing a problem with an open mind.

I am thankful to my parents who have given me full support and confidence to complete this work. I am thankful to my patients for their support and confidence in me. I am thankful to Mrs. Renu Tikku and Ms. Ranjana Chakarvarty who helped me in the artistic work of this book.

I cannot forget to thanks Dr. P.N. Jain and Mr. Kuldeep Jain who gave me this opportunity to do this project and that too in a very short sketched time.

I hope this work of mine will enlighten all of us on this big "Arthritis". In case of questions or queries contact

Dr. Ritu Arora
B-4/22 Paschim Vihar
N. Delhi - 110 063
Phone - 5583377

Contents

Contents

MORPHOLOGY AND EXAMINATION OF JOINTS

Before studying the disease, how to examine a diseased joint it is very important to understand the structural morphology and physiology of the joints.

A typical mobile free joint is shown. The bones do not touch each other but are covered by an articular cartilage which forms a cushion between the bony surfaces. At the margins of articular cartilage the **synovial membrane** is attached. This membrane is folded to allow a free joint movement. It encloses the synovial cavity and into it secretes a viscous lubricating fluid the synovial fluid.

The synovial membrane is surrounded by a fibrous joint capsule, which in turn is strengthened by ligament extending from bone to bone.

Some joints are slightly movable by vertebral bodies. Here the bones are not separated by a synovial membrane but by a fibro cartilaginous disc. At the centre of each disc is the nucleus pulposus, fibrogelatinous material that forms a cushion or a shock absorber between the vertebral bodies.

Bursae are disc shaped, fluid filled synovial sacs that occur at points of friction around and facilitate movement. They lie between the skin and the convex surface of a bone or joint or in areas where tendons or muscles rub against bone, ligaments or other tendons or muscles.

Vertebral body

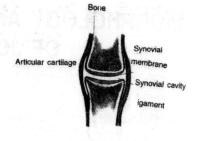

Temporomandibular joint: The temporomandibular joint forms the articulation between mandible and skull. Feel for it just in front of the tragus of each ear as the jaw is opened and closed.

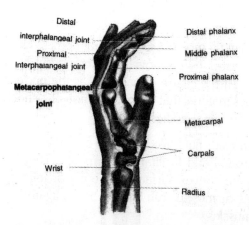

Wrist and Hands: At the wrist identify the bony tips of the radius (laterally) and the ulna (medially). On the dorsum of the wrist, palpate the groove of the radiocarpal or wrist joint.

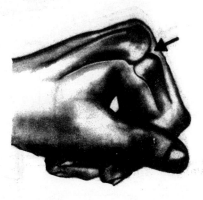

Palpate each of the five metacarpals and the proximal, middle, and distal phalanges. (The thumb lacks a middle phalanx.) Flex the hand somewhat and find the groove marking the metacarpophalangeal joint of each finger. It is distal to the knuckle and can be felt best on either side of the extensor tendon.

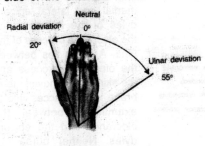

And at the joints of the fingers:

Proximal Interphalangeal Joint

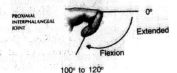

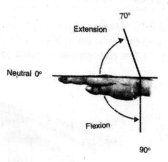

Metacarpophalangeal Joint

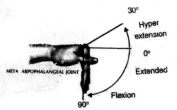

Distal Interphalangeal Joint

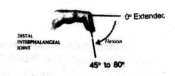

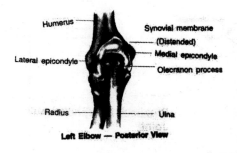

Left Elbow — Posterior View

Elbows: Identify the medial and lateral epicondyles of the humerus and the olecranon process of the ulna. A bursa lies between the olecranon process and the skin. The synovial membrane is most accessible to examination between the olecranon and the epicondyles. Neither bursa nor synovium is normally palpable, however. The sensitive ulnar nerve can be felt posteriorly between olecranon and medial epicondyle.

Movements at the elbow are illustrated below.

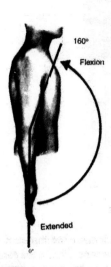

160°

Flexion

Extended

0°

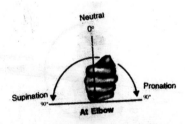

Pronation and supination of the forearm take place at the two radioulnar joints, one at the elbow and one at the wrist.

Pronation and supination of the forearm take place at the two radioulnar joints, one at the elbow and one at the wrist.

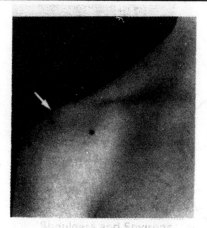

Shoulders and Environs

Rotate the arm externally and find the tendinous cord that runs just medial to the grater tubercle. Roll it under your fingers. This is the tendon of the long head of the biceps. It runs in the bicipital groove between greater and lesser tubercles.

The normal *range of motion at the shoulder is illustrated below.*

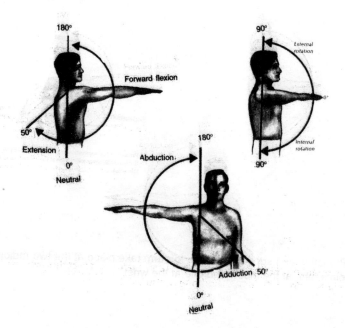

Abduction at the shoulder has two components: movement of the arm at the glenohumeral joint, and movement of the shoulder girdle (clavicle and scapula) in relation to the thorax. When one movement is restricted or painful, the other can partially compensate.

Ankles and Feet: The principal landmarks of the ankle are (1) the medial malleolus, the bony prominence at the distal end of the tibia, and (2) the lateral malleolus, the distal end of the fibula. Ligaments extend from each malleolus onto the foot. The strong Achilles tendon inserts on the heel posteriorly.

Motions *at the ankle joint* itself (the tibiotalar joint) are limited to dorsiflexion and plantar flexion.

Inversion *and eversion of the foot* are functions of the subtalar (talocalcaneal) and transverse tarsal joints.

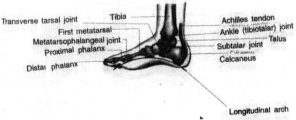

The heads of the metatarsals are palpable in the ball of the foot. These and the associated metatarsophalangeal joints are proximal to the webs of the toes. An imaginary line along the foot bones extending from the heads of the metatarsals to the calcaneus is called the longitudinal arch.

The Knee: Identify the flat medial surface of the tibia — the shin. Follow its anterior border upward to the tibial tuberosity. Mark this point with a dot of ink. Now follow the medial border of the tibia upwad until it merges into a bony prominence — the medial condyle of the tibia. This is somewhat higher than the tibial tuberosity. In a comparable location on the otherside of the knee, find a similar prominence — the lateral condyle. Mark both condyles with ink.

With the knee flexed about 90° you can press your thumbs — one on each side of the patellar tendon — into the groove of the tibiofemoral joint. Note that the patella lies just above this joint line. As you press downward you can feel the edges of the tibial plateaus, the upper surfaces of the tibia.

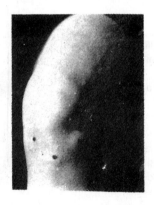

Pelvis and hips: The hip joint lies deep and is not directly palpable. The greater trochanter of the femur can be felt about a palm's breadth below the iliac crest. The superficial trochanteric bursa lies on the posterolateral surface of the greater trochanter.

The principal *movements of the knee* are extension, flexion, and sometimes hyperextension.

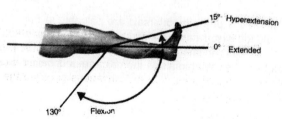

With knee straight   **With knee flexed**

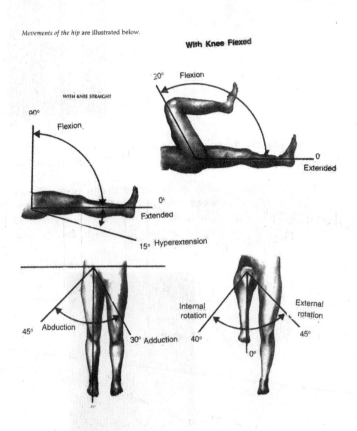

Movements of the hip are illustrated below.

Spine: Viewing the patient from behind, identify the following landmarks: (1) the spinous processes, which become more evident on forward flexion, (2) the paravertebral muscles on either side of the midline, (3) the scapula, (4) the iliac crests, and (5) the posterior superior iliac spines, usually marked by skin dimples. The spinous processes of C7 and often T1 are usually prominent. A line between the iliac crests crosses the spinous process of L4

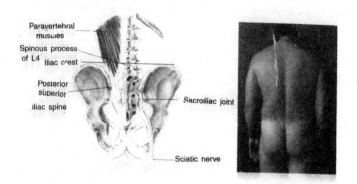

Viewed laterally, the spine has cervical and lumbar concavities and a thoracic convexity. The sacral curve forms a second convexity.

The most mobile portion of the spine is the neck. Flexion and extension occur chiefly between the head and the 1st cervical vertebra, rotation occurs primarily between the 1st and 2nd vertebrae, and lateral bending involves the cervical spine from the 2nd to the 7th vertebra.

Cervical concavity

Thoracic convexity

Lumbar concavity

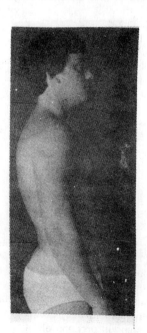

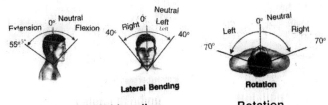

Lateral bending   Rotation

Movements of the rest of the spine (i.e., from the sacrum to the base of the neck) are more difficult to measure than those in the neck and are subject to considerable individual variation. What looks like spinal flexion takes place partly at the hips. For this reason, and because people differ in the length of their estimated by noting the distance of their fingertips from the floor. As the patient flexes forward, watch the lumbar area. Its normal convavity should flatten out

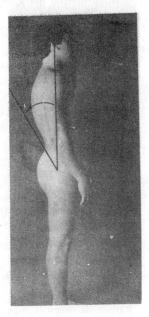

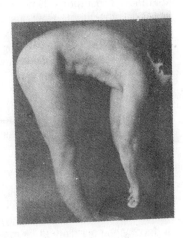

Flexion

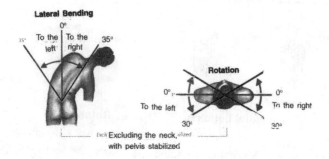

Lateral Bending

To the left | To the right

Rotation

To the left   To the right

Excluding the neck,
with pelvis stabilized

Lateral bending

Rotation

Techniques of Examination

While examining the musculoskeletal system, direct your attention not only to structure but also to function.

In your initial survey of the patient you have assessed general appearance, bodily proportions, and ease of movement. Now, using inspection and palpation, you will examine individual joints or groups of joints, their range of motion, and the tissues surrounding them.

Note particularly:

1. *Any limitation* in the normal *range of motion* or any unusual increase in the mobility of the joint.

2. Any signs of inflammation such as:

a. Swelling in or around the joint. Swelling may involve the synovial membrane, which then feels boggy, or doughy, to your gingers, or may be produced by excessive synovial fluid within the joint space.

b. Tenderness in or around the joint. Try to define the specific anatomic structure that is tender.

Decreased range of motion in arthritis, inflammation of tissues around the joint, fibrosis in or around a joit, or bony fixation (ankylosis)

Palpable bogginess, or doughiness, of the synovial membrane indicates synovitis. Palpable joint fluid indicates an effusion in the joint. Synovitis and joint fluid often coexist.

Arthritis, tendonitis, bursitis, osteomyelitis.

Tenderness and warmth over a thickened synovium suggest rheumatoid arthritis.

Redness of the skin over a tender joint suggests septic or goity arthritis, or possibly rheumatic fever.

Fine, soft crepitus may be felt over inflamed joints. Coarser crepitus suggests roughened articular cartilages, a sin an inflamed joint or osteoarthritis. A

c. Increased heat. Use the backs of your finges to compare the joint with the symmetrical joint on the opposite side or, if both joints are involved, with the tissues near them.

Redness of the overlying skin.

3. Crepitus (crepitation), a palpable or even audible crunching or grating produced by movement of a joint or tendon. Crepitus is more significant when it is associated with other symptoms or signs than when it exists by itself. Cracking or snapping sounds, which result from movement of tendons or ligaments over bone, may occur in normal joints such as the knees.

4. Deformities, including:

   Malalignment of articulating bones

   An abnormality in the relationship between two articulating surfaces

5. The condition of the surrounding tissues, including muscle atrophy, subcutaneous nodules, and skin changes.

6. Muscular strength.

7. Symmetry of involvement. Note whether arthritic changes involve several joints symmetrically on both sides of the body or afffect only one or perhaps two joints.

creaking leathery crepitus may arise in inflamed tendon sheaths.

Flexion deformity of the hip.

Ulnar deviation of the fingers in rheumatoid arthritis .

Dislocation, a complete loss of contact between the two surfaces, and subluxation, a partial loss of contact.

Suncutaneous nodules in rheumatoid arthritis or rheumatic fever.

Muscular weakness and atrophy in rheumatoid arthritis.

Involvement of only one joint increases the likelihood of bacterial arthritis. Rheumatoid arthritis typically involves several joints, symmertically distributed.

Scoliosis is an important problem in adolescents, especially girls, and is frequently asymptomatic in its early stages.

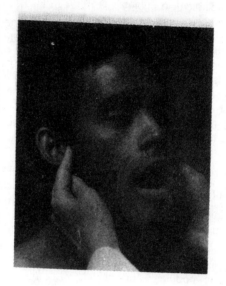

With the patient sitting up

Head and neck

To palpate the temporomandibular joint, place the tip of your index finger just in front of the tragus of each ear and ask the patient to open the mouth. The tips of your fingers should drop into the joint spaces as the mouth opens. Observe the range of motion, feel for swelling, and note any tenderness. Snapping or clicking may be felt and heard in normal people.

Inspect the neck for defrmities and abnormal posture.

Palpate the spinous processes of the cervical spine and the related soft tissues, including the trapezius muscles, the muscles between the scapulae, and the sternomastoids. Identify any areas of tenderness.

Test the range of motion by asking the patient to:

Touch chin to chest (flexion)

Touch chin to each shoulder (rotation)

Touch each ear to the corresponding shoulder without raising the shoulder (lateral bending)

Put the head back (extension)

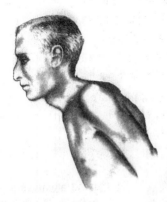

Hands and Wrists

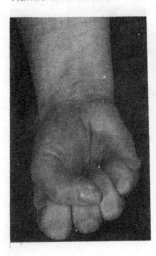
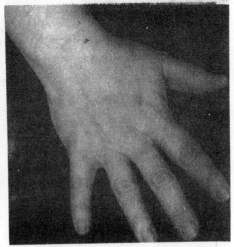

Test the range of motion of the fingers and wrists by asking the patient to:

1. Make a fist with each hand, thumb across the knuckles, and then extend and spread the fingers.

A person should be able to make tight fists and extend and spread the fingers smoothly and easily.

Conditions that impair range of motion include arthritis, inflammation of the tendon sheaths (tenosynovitis), and fibrosis in the palmar fascia Duptuyren's contracture).

2. Flex and extend the wrists, and with palms down turn the hands laterally and medially (ulnar and radial deviation). Because grip is strongest when the wrist is partly extended, impaired extension is especially important.

Inspect the hands and wrists, noting any swelling, redness, nodules, deformity or muscular atrophy.

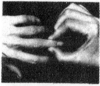

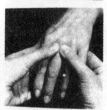

Palpate the medial and lateral aspects of each interphalangeal joint between your thumb and index finger, noting any swelling, bogginess, bony enlargement, or tenderness.

With your thumbs palpate the metacarpophalangeal joints, just distal to and on each side of the knuckle.

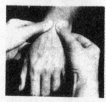

Palpate each wrist joint, with your thumbs on the dorsum of the wrist, your fingers beneath it. Note any swelling, bogginess, or tenderness.

Osteoarthritis of the distal interphalangeal joint appears as hard dorsolateral nodules called Herberden's nodes.

The proximal interphalangeal joints are affected less often. Rheumatoid arthritis commonly involves the proximal joints.

Rheumatoid arthritis often involves the metacarpophalangeal joints; osteoarthritis rarely does.

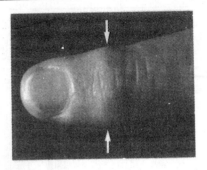

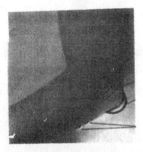

Elbows

Test the range of motion by asking the patient to bend and straighten the elbows.

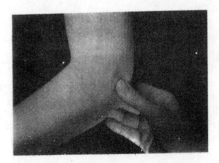

Support the patient's forearm with your opposite hand so that the elbow is flexed to about 70°. Inspect and palpate the elbow, including theextensor surface of the ulna and the olecranon process, noting any nodules or swelling.

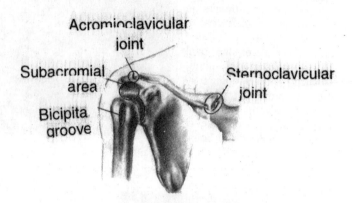

Acromioclavicular joint

Subacromial area

Bicipital groove

Sternoclavicular joint

Shoulders
The most common cause of shoulder pain is rotator cuff tendinitis

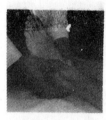

Ankles and Feet
Look for rheumatoid nodules; tenderness of achilles tendinitis or bursitis

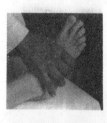

Tenderness on compression of the metatarsophalangeal joints is an early sign of rheumatoid arthritis. Acute inflammation of the first metatarsophalangeal joint suggests gout.

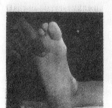

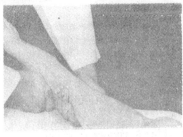 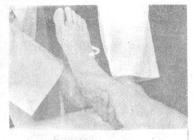

Inversion   **Eversion**

An arthritic joint is frequently painful when moved in any direction, while a ligamenttous sprain produces maximal pain when the ligament is stretched.

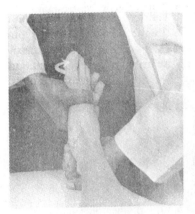 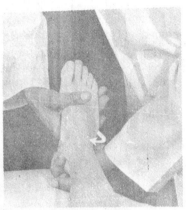

Inversion   **Eversion**

Knees and Hips: Inspect the knees, noting their alignment and any deformity. Note any atrophy of the quadriceps muscles. Look for loss of the normal hollows around the patella (an early sign of swelling in the knee joint and suprapatellar pouch), and note any other swelling in or around the knee.

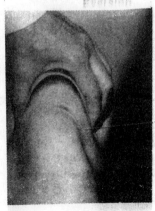

Suprapatellar pouch

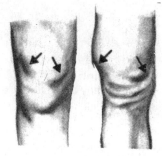

Swelling above and adjacent to the patella suggests synovial thickening or fluid in the knee joint.

Thickening bogginess, tenderness, and warmth in these areas indicates synovial inflammation. Nontender effusions are common in osteoarthritis.

Bursitis causes a more localized swelling, as in prepatellar bursitis (housemaid's knee).

Moderate swelling   **Marked swelling**

A bulge of returning fluid indicates an effusion with the knee joint.

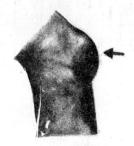

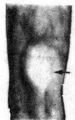
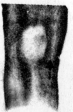
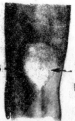

← Swelling

Press ← Swelling reappea

Milk upward

Milk upward
Look for a bulge sign.
1. With the ball of your hand milk the medial aspect of the knee firmly upward two or three times to displace any fluid

2. Then press or tap the knee just behind the lateral margin of the patella

Try to Ballotte a "Floating patella": Firmly grasp the thigh just above the patella with one hand, thus forcing fluid out of the suprepatellar pouch into the space between the patella and femur. With the fingers of your other hand, push the patella sharply back against the femur. Feel for a palpable tap. In the absence of fluid none is felt because the patella is already snug against the femur.

Apply manual pressure here
to displace knee fluid   Briskly tap here to click the
into space behind   patella against the femur.
patella

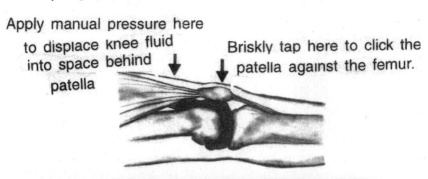

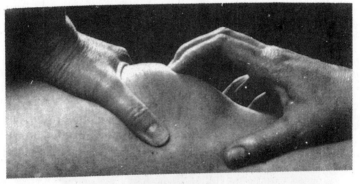

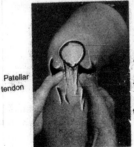

Patella

Lateral
epicondyle

Patellar   Lateral collateral
tendon   Tibia   ligament

Tibial
tuberosity

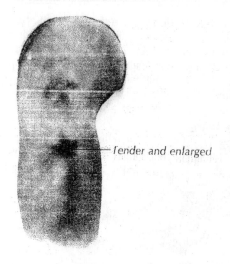

A tender, swollen tibial tuberosity in an adolescent suggests Osgood - Schlatter disease.

Tender and enlarged

Range of Motion at knees and hips. Ask the patient to bend each knee in turn up to the chest and pull it firmly against the abdomen.

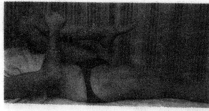

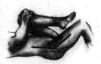

Flexion of the opposite thigh indicates a flexion deformity of that hip.

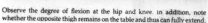

Observe the degree of flexion at the hip and knee. In addition, note whether the opposite thigh remains on the table and thus can fully extend.

Flexion of the opposite thigh indicates a flexion deformity of that hip. Restriction of internal rotation is an especially sensitive indicator of hip disease such as arthritis. External rotation is often restricted also.

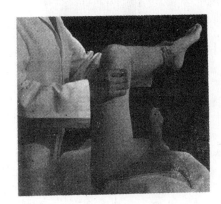

External Rotation

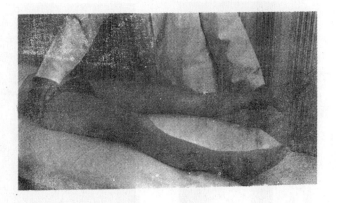

Alternatively, stand at the foot of the table, grasp both ankles, and abduct both extended legs at the hips

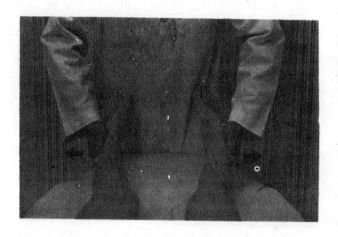

This method allows easy comparison of the two sides when movements are restricted.

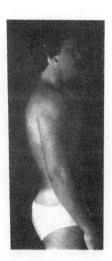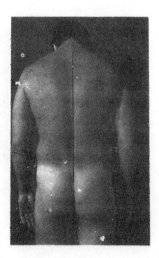

The spine: The gown should allow adequate visualization of the patient's spine.

From the side inspect the spinal profile, noting the cervical, thoracic, and lumbar curves.

From behind the patient inspect the spine for lateral curves. Look for any differences in the heights of the shoulders, the iliac crests, and the skin creases below the buttocks. Note whether an imaginary line dropped from the spinous process of T1 falls, as it should, through the gluteal creft.

Sit down, stabilize the patient's pelvis with your hands, and ask the patient to (1) bend sideways (lateral bending), (2) bend backwards toward you (extension), and (3) twist the shoulders one way and then the other (rotation).

From a sitting or standing position, palpate the spinous processes with your thumb. In the lower lumbar area determine whether one spinous process seems unusually prominent in relation to the one above it. Identify any tenderness.

You may also wish to percuss the spine for tenderness by thumping it (not too roughly) with the ulnar surface of your fist.

Inspect and palpate the paravertebral muscles for tenderness and spasm. Palpate for tenderness in any other areas that are suggested by the patient's symptoms. Try to identify the underlying structures involved. A skin dimple usually overlies the posterior iliac spine and guides you onward the sacroiliac area.

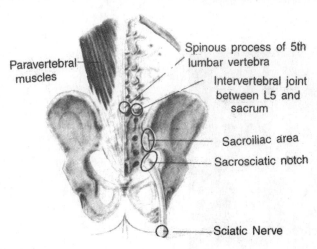

Paravertebral muscles

Spinous process of 5th lumbar vertebra

Intervertebral joint between L5 and sacrum

Sacroiliac area

Sacrosciatic notch

Sciatic Nerve

See pages 456–457 for further testing of low back pain with leg radiation

Herniated intervertebral discs, most common between L5 and S1 or between L4 and L5, may produce tenderness of the spinous processes, the intervertebral joints, the paravertebral muscles, the sacrosciatic notch, and the sciatic nerve.

Rheumatoid arthritis may also cause tenderness of the intervertebral joints. Ankylosing spondylitis may produce sacroiliac tenderness.

Phalen's Test. Hold the patient's wrists in acute flexion for 60 seconds. Alternatively, ask the patient to press the back of both hands together to form right angles.

If numbness and tingling develop over the distribution of the median nerve (e.g., the palmar surface of the thumb, and the index, middle, and part of the ring fingers) the sign is positive, suggesting the carpal tunnel syndrome.

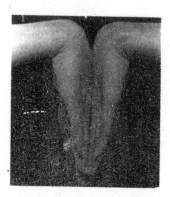

If numbness and tingling develop over the distribution of the median nerve (*e.g.*, the palmar surface of the thumb, and the index, middle, and part of the ring fingers) the sign is positive, suggesting the carpal tunnel syndrome.

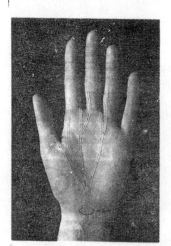

Tingling or electric sensations in the distribution of the median nerve constitute a positive test, suggesting the carpal tunnel syndrome.

Tinel's Sign. With your finger percuss lightly over the course of the median nerve in the carpal turnel at the spot indicated by the arrow.

Tingling or electric sensations in the distrubution of the median nerve constitute a positive test, suggesting the carpal tunnel syndrome

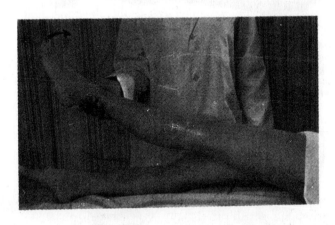

Measuring the length of legs. If you suspect that the patient's legs are unequal in length, measure them. Get the patient relaxed in the supine position and symmetrically aligned with legs extended. With a tape, measure the distance between anterior superior iliac spine and the medial malleolus. The tape should cross the knee on its medial side.

Sharp pain radiating from the back down the leg in an L5 or S1 distribution (radicular pain) suggests tension or compression of the nerve root(s), often caused by a herniated lumbar disc. Dorsiflexion of the foot increases the pain. Increased pain in the affected leg when the opposite leg is raised strongly confirms radicular parin and constitutes a positive *crossed straight leg - raising sign.*

Describing limited motion of a joint: Although precise measurement of motion is not routinely necessary, limitations can be described in degrees. Pocket goniometers are available for this purpose. In the two examples shown below the dark lines indicate the range of the patient's movement and the black lines show the normal range.

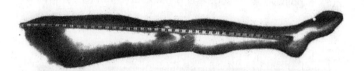

DESCRIBING LIMITED MOTION OF A JOINT. Although precise measurement of motion is not routinely necessary, limitations can be described in degrees. Pocket goniometers are available for this purpose. In the two examples shown below, the red lines indicate the range of the patient's movement and the black lines show the normal range.

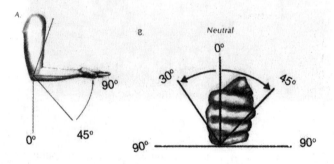

A. The elbow flexes from 45° 90° (45° - 90°)
- or -

The elbow has a flexion deformity of 45° and flexes farther to 90o (45° - 90°)
B. Supination at elbow = 30°)0° - 30°)
Pronation at elbow = 45° (0° - 45°)

CLASSIFICATION OF ARTHRITIS

Although arthritis has a wide variety of presentations but it can be simply classified into acute, subacute and chronic groups depending primarily on the presentation, course and prognosis of illness.

ARTHRITIS

Acute | **Subacute** | **Chronic**

Acute
a. Acute Rheumatism.
b. Acute Gout.
c. Reiter's Disease.
   (Gonococcal arthritis)

d. Acute rheumatoid arthritis.
e. Acute suppurative arthritis.
f. Acute specific fevers.
g. Extension from adjacent bones.

Chronic
1. Osteoarthritis.
2. Chronic R.A.

3. Chronic gonococcal arthritis.
4. Chronic Gout.
5. Ankylosing spondylitis.
6. Chronic infective arthritis.
7. S.L.E.
8. Syphilitic arthritis.
9. Polyarteritis Nodosa.
10. Neuro pathic arthritis.

Criteria for acute arthritis: Acute onset is abrupt, sudden with general and local signs of inflammation and associated septicaemia. It is usually an erratic poly arthritis which affects one joint primarily. It is primarily due to some infective process or some underlying systemic. disorders. It needs immediate attention and correction of cause underneath.

Criteria of chronic arthritis: They have an insidious onset with a slow progress but a definite tendency to destruct the tissues gradually. It is progressive in nature and leads to destruction of articular and periarticular tissues.

We shall be studying every type of arthritis in details in the coming chapters. Every arthritis has been discussed in terms of

a. General presentations.

b. Etiology

c. Signs and symptoms

d. Diagnosis

e. Prognosis

f. Treatment

g. Associated symptoms or secondary manifestations.

h. Differential diagnosis if any.

RHEUMATOID ARTHRITIS

General introduction: Rheumatoid arthritic is one of the very commonest auto immune disorders which has it's systemic presentations affecting both articular and para articular tissues. This auto immune disease has a significant resemblance to the protean group of acquired diseases in which genetic factors play an important role.

Etiology: The exact etiology is unknown: But persons with HLA, DWR suggest a genetic predisposition. It is generally a symmetrical, polyarthritis which is characterised by both articular and non articular lesions.

Pathology:

1. Synovium shows fibrinoid degeneration. Surrounded by infiltration with fibroblasts and mononuclear infilterates.

Synovial membrane becomes thickend hyperemic and oedomatous.

2. Later vascular proliferations invades the articular cartilage to form a pannus. It leads to destruction of articular cartilage.

Signs & Symptoms:

1. It affects females primarily in the age group of 20 years to 45 years.

2. Prodromal symptoms are excessive fatigue, transient loss of weight. Initially occasional presentation of capsulitis shoulder or a heel pain is the indication.

3. **Arthritic symptoms:** Start in different ways

    a. Affecting 2nd and 3rd fingers of proximal I.P. joints of fingers, gradually affecting metacarpophalangeal joints.

    b. It is followed by pain and swelling of knees, shoulders, ankles and lately hip joints also.

4. **Constitutional symptoms:** Usually generalised malaise with low grade fever or moderate fever, weight loss and anaemia.

    Extra-articular manifestations: It affects the systems other than joints.

1. **Skin:** Painless, non tender nodules. Mainly subcutaneous are seen. Raynaud's phenomenon, vasculitis of nail, palmar erythema, hyperhidrosis of extremities, non healing ulcers are few manifestations.

2. **Eyes:** a. Scleritis is the most commonest presentation. In necrotising sclerosis, nodules degenerate and impart a deep blue colour. It may even present as scleromalacia perforans ie. preforation of sclera.

3. **Respiratory manifestations** a. Dyspnoea b. Stridor or laryngismus stridulus is also one of the manifestations c. Recurrent pleural effusion. d. Caplan's syndrome: It occurs in combination of R.A. with repeat pneumoconinosis, demonstrable nodules in lung fields seen on X-ray.

4. **Cardio vascular:** It includes pericarditis, aortic regurgitation and conduction defects.

5. **Neuropathy:** a. Carpal tunnel syndrome b. Symmetrical neuropathy. c. In severe cases foot drop, wrist drop may develop.

6. **Metabolic presentations:** Secondary amyloidosis is one of the presentations.

Clinical signs of R.A.: 1. Fusiform, spindle shaped lesions at I.P. joints, metacarpophalangeal joints.

2. Patchy hyperpigmentation or freckles on face.

3. Rheumatoid nodules underneath skin.

Diagnosis: It is of 2 types.

a. **Clinical Diagnosis:** It aims at looking for the very early clinical manifestations which is helped by the good observations of the physician. The constitutional look of face, colour of skin, any nodes may help.

b. **Laboratory diagnosis:** a. E.S.R. is moderately to severely raised.

   b. Confirmed positive R.A. Factor, C-RP protein.

c. Hypochromic, microcytic anaemia.

d. **Serology:** Igm, can be demonstrated by rose waaler test, latex fixation test.

e. **Synovial fluid aspiration:** In arthritis it reveals a turbid fluid of low viscosity and poor mucinclot. The W.B.C. count increases beyond 1500. Cumm. The protein content is quite high.

f. **X-ray:** In the initial stage changes are seen either in wrist or ankle joints with soft tissue swelling erosions seen at I.P. joints with gradual space reduction.

Radiologically the lesions have been graded into.

1. **Grade I:** Soft tissue swelling with or without juxta articular osteoporosis.

2. **Grade II:** Narrowing of joint space due to cartilage destruction.

3. **Grade III:** Erosions, either surface or cystic erosions.

4. **Grade IV:** Marked irregularity of articular surfaces with subluxations and secondary degenerative changes.

Diagnostic criteria: According to American rheumatic association if out of the following characteristics, the scoring is 7/11 it is a classical rheumatoid arthritis. If the scoring is 5/11 it is termed as definite rheumatoid arthritis. And if it is 3/11 it is probable rheumatoid arthritis.

The term possible rheumatoid arthritis indicates the presence of any one of the following.

a. Morning stiffness.

b. Pain and tenderness of joints.

c. History of joint swelling observed by the physician.

d. High ESR.

e. Subcutaneous nodules.

American criteria are:

1. Morning stiffness of nearly 1/2 hour duration.

2. Positive rose waaler test.

3. Symmetrical swelling of identical joints except distal I.P. joints.

4. X-ray changes.

5. Poor mucin clot in synovial fluid.

6. Subcutaneous nodules.

7. Pain or tenderness in at least one joint.

8. Biopsy evidence in the nodules.

9. Swelling of one other joint as observed by the physician with a 3 month interval between the appearance of 2 joint swellings

10. Swelling of at least one joint as observed by a physician.

11. Histology of synovial membrane showing at least 3 of the features

   a. Villious hypertrophy.

   b. Lymph follicle formation.

   c. Fibrinoid necrosis.

   d. Foci of cell necrosis.

Differential diagnosis: It should be differentiated from

   a. Rheumatic arthritis.

   b. Psoriatic arthritis.

   c. Reiter's syndrome.

Prognosis: In general it has a tendency to recur with acute exacerbations. It leads to progressive deformity and disability. The favourable criteria are

   a. Acute onset.

   b. Male sex.

   c. Onset at late age.

   d. A symmetrical or monoarticular involvement.

   e. Negative rheumatoid factor.

   f. Prompt response to therapy.

Treatment: 1. General management:

   a. Giving rest.

b. Give plenty of fluids.

c. Reduce muscle spasm.

2. Specific treatment: a. Medication for constitutional symptoms. b. Physiotherapy which includes paraffin wax, ultrasonic etc.

There are different variants of rheumatoid arthritis.

1. **Chronic Juvenile polyarthritis:** It starts before the age of 16 years. It affects primarily females and is associated with rash fever, lymphadenopathy and spleeno meagly. Eye complications with keratopathy and uveitis are common.

2. **Felty's syndrome:** It is seen in the elderly age group and is featured with positive rheumatoid factor, spleenomeagly and neutropenia.

3. **Sjogren's syndrome:** It consists of keratoconjunctivitis Sicca, seropositive rheumatoid arthritis and xerostomia. It is also known as sicca syndrome.

4. **Palindromic rheumatism:** In this repeated attacks of joint pains occur with redness and swelling but without any residual lesions. It is followed by typical rheumatoid features.

RHEUMATIC ARTHRITIS

General arthritis:

General Introduction: Acute. Rheumatism is mainly a disease of temperate climates. It is not seen before 4 years of the and is rare after 25 years the attacks are more common in winters.

Etiology: (a) Cause is β Haemolytic streptococcal infection with a history of tonsillitis.

Signs and symptoms:

1. A continued type of fever comes lasting for 3-4 days. It is accompanied by septic features of quick, bounding pulse, coated tongue and high coloured scanty urine.

2. It is followed by profuse perspiration which has a sour, disagreeable taste with an acidic reaction.

3. Wandering joint pains with inflammation. Joints are highly painful, aggravated on slightest touch and by movement.

4. Cardiac symptom in the form of mild discomfort with a pericardial Rub is heard

5. Early signs of mitral endocarditis appears.

6. Rheumatic nodules may or may not appear.

7. Occasionally chorea may be the only sign of presentation.

Diagnosis

1. Raised E.S.R. and ASO titre.

2. Throat culture isolates β haemolytic streptococcus.

ACUTE AND CHRONIC GOUT

General introduction: It is a purine metabolic disorder resulting in hyperuricemia with the deposits of urate crystals in the synovium and clinically manifesting as recurrent acute arthritis progressing to chronic deforming arthritis with a formation of gouty tophi. The term gout usually indicates a heterogenous group of diseases characterised by hyperurecemia.

Etiology: The normal plasma level is between 2-7 mg/dl. The causes can be categorised into:

a. **Primary:** It is the most importants cause which means either overproduction or underexcretion of uric acid.

1. **Secondary:** It indicates the presence of some demonstrable disorder which leads either to overproduction or defective excretion of uric acid.

Causes are:

1. Excessive breakdown due to overmedication eg. in leukaemia, myeloma etc.

2. **Inborn errors of metabolism** eg. Type-I glycogen storage diseases.

3. **Lesch nyhan syndrome:** In this deficiency of hypoxanthene glianine, phosphoribosyl transferae is absent.

3. Impaired excretion in: a. Chronic renal failure b. Lactic acidosis c. Intake of drugs.

Prognosis: It is usually good. But sometimes it may lead to endocarditis, myocarditis, rarely pneumonitis.

Differential diagnosis: a.Meningo coccal septicaemia

b. Lymphatic leukaemia c. Gonococcal arthritis d. Infective endocarditis.

Treatment: 1. It includes rest and managing the general constitutional symptoms.

2. Treat the throat infection.

3. Use of analgesics is indicated. Thiazides, salicylates etc.

Clinical symptoms:

1. Symptoms of an acute attack are preceded by Dyspepsia, aching in the limbs, with pain in the middle of night.

2. Joints are painful, throb to touch. It is followed by perspiration which slightly relieves.

3. The attack is usually precipitated by alcohol bouts, infections, dietary excess, undue physical exercise, surgery and withdrawl of drugs.

4. In chronic gout the affected joints are painful with gouty tophi painful tender joints.

5. Subcutaneous nodules which are hard. They are found in the tendo achillis, helix of ears.

Diagnosis. a. High ESR, high levels of uric acid are the 1st indications. b. Radiological evidence shows small punched out erosions due to urate deposits.

Prognosis: It is fairly good but has a tendency to increase fairly.

Treatment:

1. Rest to the part.

2. Correction of the underlying cause.

3. Cut off totally a very high protein intake and increase the water content.

4. Need of analgesics to relieve pain

PSEUDO GOUT

First indicates the acute intermittent arthritis caused by the deposition of Calcium pyrophosphate dihydrate in the synovium. The crystals are seen in the articular synovium.

OSTEOARTHRITIS

General introduction: It is usually a chronic degenerative disease of joints progressive in nature occurring mainly in the middle half of life. It may affect one joint or many joints but usually seen above 40 years of age.

Etiology: It is caused primarily by wear and tear to the joints. The causes can be primary or secondary. Presence and absence of hebreden's nodes help in identifying the type of disease.

1. Hereditary factors.

2. Ageing process.

3. Overuse of joints.

4. Secondary causes include.

   a. Preexisting joint disease.

   b. Endocrine disorders like diabetes, acromeagly, hyper parathyroidism, sensory neuropathies.

   c. Hypermobility seen in charcot's joints.

   d. Obesity.

   e. Orthopediac deformities.

Pathology: Due to mechanical stress, the collagen fibre network of the articular cartilage is disrupt. It leads to alteration in the composition of ground connective tissue with resultant loss of resillience.

The chondocytes increase thus leading to further disruption of collagen tissues. Synovial fluid gains access to the deeper layers of cartilage. It adds to further destruction of weight bearing cartilage.

Signs and symptoms:

1. Onset is gradual and can be seen in either sex usually above 40 years of age. It affects primarily the weight bearing joints of hips, knees, shoulders etc.

2. Pain is felt after exercise and after a period of immobility. Pain is aching, initially it is, intermittent then becomes continuous.

3. Stiffness is the first symptoms while getting up in the morning.

4. Gradually all movements are restricted and it may lead to complete inability to walk and perform normal life activities.

5. Hebreden's nodes at the distal I.P. joints is the clinical · indication.

6. Scrunching and grating are audible and gradually may be felt by the patient.

7. Considerable deformities may occur due to muscle spasm.

8. Radiological evidence shows sub chondrial sclerosis, narrowing of joint space, joint destruction, osteophyte formation, cystic formation in joints with presence of loose bodies in the joint space.

MANAGEMENT AND TREATMENT:

1. Prevention of over use of affected joints.

2. Limitation of activity to reduce pain

3. Application of heat and graded movements.

4. Physiotherapy and classical acupuncture are highly useful.

MENOPAUSAL ARTHRITIS

It is a small group of arthritis which occurs in women between 40 and 50 yrs of age. It mainly involves the knees and occasionally wrists and fingers. It usually presents with all the features of osteoarthritis but a mild feature of inflammation is associated in menopausal group of arthritis.

GENERAL MANAGEMENT

1. It aims at correcting the cause of menopause in the background.

2.   In this homoeopathic management is clinically very useful.

3.   Osteoporosis may develop so iron and calcium intake should be maintained.

GONOCOCCAL ARTHRITIS

It is now a lesser forms of arthritis. It is usually related to the gonococcal infection and may take years together to present the symptoms.

Etiology: It is usually found in the young and middle age group when the focus of infection is in the urethra or prostate in male and cervix or uterus in females usually resembling other forms of infective arthritis.

Clinical signs and symptoms:

1.   It affects primarily the big joints of knees, ankles, elbows, shoulders etc.

2.   Affected joints are painful, red, hot.

3.   Moderate fever is usually associated.

4.   Tendo achilles is sometimes painful.

5.   Periostitis or iridocyclitis may occur.

Diagnosis:

1.   Leucocytosis.

2.   High E.S.R.

3.   Positive complement fixation test for gonococci.

Prognosis: It is usually a short lasting arthritis with a limited period of infection.

Treatment: Of underlying cause if essential.

TUBERCULAR ARTHRITIS

General introduction: It affects primarily the synovial membrane but occasionally it may start in the articular ends of bones. It is a mono articular joint affection seen mainly in children.

Signs and symptoms:

1. Onset is slow and date back to history of injury.
2. It affects primarily the hip joint and knees.
3. Usually constitutional symptoms with malaise, low grade fever are present.

    Treatment: 1. It needs good diet, sunlight, fresh, open air.

    2. Treatment of cause by antitubercular medicine.

SYPHILITIC JOINT DISEASE

It is also one of the manifestations where secondary stage of syphillis is usually associated with subacute arthritis affecting only one joint.

1. The joints are comparatively painless with restricted movement but a doughy touch of joint.
2. Pains are more at night with or without low grade temperature.
3. In rare cases pseudo paralysis of syphilitic origin occurs leading to complications.

HYSTERICAL JOINTS

It is usually seen in hypersensitive nervous, hysterical females who show the features of muscle stiffness and immobility. It usually affects knee or hip with a history of grief or mental trauma.

The joints are usually normal to touch but with a marked muscle spasm.

NEUROPATHIC JOINTS

In the diseases of spinal column namely tabes dorsalis and syringomylia these joint disorders are associated. There is extensive degeneration of joints with complete lack of flexibility. It is fully mobile and can be hyperextended or flexed. In all these cases pupils are dilated and knee and ankle jerks should be assessed, they are exaggerated.

PSORIATIC ARTHRITIS

General introduction:

It is also covered under autoimmune group which is characterised by nail changes of psoriasis associated with involvements of metatarso phalangeal joints. Rose waaler test gives a negative response.

Systemic lupus erythematosis: (S.L.E.) It is an inflammatory disease of autoimmune nature involving the connective tissue of several organ systems.

Etiology:

1. It is predominantly seen in females. It results from severe immune disturbances, with the production of several auto immune antibodies and complexes.

2. Genetic factors play an important role.

3. Drugs and viral infections may precipitate.

Pathology: The lesions lead to

    a. Fibrinoid necrosis

    b. Collagen sclerosis

c. Formation of haematoxylon bodies

d. Inflammatory changes in arterioles and capillaries.

Tissue damage occurs due to

a. Direct cytotoxicity

b. Type III immune reaction.

Clinical features: It is more prevalent in females in the age group of 2nd and third decade. The symptoms are:

1. **Arthritis and arthralgia:** Larger joints are affected

2. **Skin lesions:** It is usually characterised by butterfly rash, specially on cheeks and nose, frontal baldness with alopecia may develop. Painful oral and pharyngeal ulcers may develop.

3. **Cardiovascular system:** They include myocarditis, pericardial effusion, valvulitis.

4. **Respiratory system:** Common lesions are dry pleurisy, fibrosing alveolitis, lupus pneumonitis, pleural effusion etc.

5. **Kidneys:** It may lead to proteinuria, haematuria, or even acute nephritis may be precipitated.

6. **C.N.S.** convulsions, psychosis, neuropathy, myelopathy with cerebellar ataxia may develop as few complications.

7. **Muscles:** Myalgia, occasionally poly myositis with muscle wasting may develop.

8. **Haemotology:** It induces hypochromic anaemia, coomb's positive hemolytic anaemia.

Diagnosis

1. Raised E.S.R.

2. Moderate anaemia with leucopenia and thrombo cytopenia are the indicators.

3. L.E. cell phenomenon is positive.

Management:

1. It aims at avoidance of recurrence and relapses.

2. Avoid direct sun light.

3. Give the appropriate medicines.

ANKYLOSING SPONDYLITIS

General introduction: It is also known as marie striumpell disease,

Ankylopoetica or Rheumatoid spondylitis. It is an inflammatory disease affecting various joints mainly of spine associated with calcification and ossification of ligaments and capsules leading to bony ankylosis.

Etiology:

1. Commonly seen in males. The ratio is 7:3.

2. HLA B27 is positive in 90% cases.

3. Genitourinary diseases are associated with this.

Pathology: It primarily affects the S.I. joints and vertebral joints. But others like symphysis affected the joints show mild synovitis, periarticular fibrosis, ligament inflammation.

Ankylosis develops in the joints leads to ossification affecting the vertebral borders leading to bamboo spine or ankylosed spine.

Signs and symptoms:

1. Initially low back pain which gradually progresses and stiffness aggravated in the morning.

2. Gradually wasting is seen and the back starts getting fixed.

3. It may also lead to atlanto axial dislocation.Compression syndrome

4.   Cardiac manifestations include aortic incompetence, atrio ventricular and intraventricular defects.

Investigations:

1.   High E.S.R. with normochronic normocytic anaemia.
2.   H.L.A. B27 +ve.
3.   Negative test for RA Factor.
4.   X-ray in early stages shows irregularity of joint margin with osteoporosis at the early page.

Treatment:

1.   Physiotherapy with rehabilitation is advisable.
2.   Osteotomy if indicated is advisable.
3.   Control the acute exacerbation of disease.

RARE FORMS OF ARTHRITIS

1.   **Viral arthritis:** It is of viral origin and usually of a short, fulminating type. It is polyarticular with a symmetrical distribution. It is usually associated with viral hepatits type B. It is tested by hepatitis surface 'B' antigen.

2.   **Arthritis in sarcoidosis:** It is rarely seen. Onset is gradual with the manifestation of knee and ankles being affected. Arthritis is never associated with destruction.

3.   **Bechcet's syndrome:** It is characterised by recurrent oral and genital ulcers, urethritis erythema nodosa, thrombo phlebitis.

4.   **Wegner's granulomatosis:** It is a rare disorder characterised by vasculitis, necrotizing granulomatosis lesions of upper and lower extremities.

Non specific arthritis

It Includes:

1. Plantar fascitis
2. Olecranon bursitis
3. Tennis elbow
4. Golfer's elbow.
5. Calcanean spur.
6. Duptyren's contracture.

Cervical Spondylosis

It is one of the most commonest degenerating disorders affecting primarily the imtervertibral discs and posterial I.V. joints. It is characterised mainly by both sensory and motor symptoms.

Etiology: Although the exact cause is unknown but there are certain factors which precipitate it

a. Excessive physical and mental stress.
b. Trauma.
c. Faulty posture

It is found in either sex and age is also not a consideration.

Clinical symptoms: It presents predominantly with

a. **Pain:** It may be either severe or even vague usually precipitated by physical stress and strain.
b. **Stiffness:** Easly morning stiffness is very well marked which gradually reduces as other activities are restored gradually.
c. **Radiating smptoms:** It usually indicates compression symoptoms which include.

1. Radiating pains along the couse of affected nerve.
2. Pain << by cough, snezing or tendency for dislocation rarely.
3. Numbness and paraesthesia with tingling in hands

d. In the late stages:

1. Severe osteoporotic changes may precipitate subluxation of intervetebral joints.

Signs on Examination:

a. Cervical spasm with or without muscle wasting.

b. Tenderness neck with restriction of movements.

Investigations:

1. E.S.R. is mildly raised.
2. X-ray shows either cervical spasm, straightening of cervical curve or reduction of intervertebral discs.
3. Osteophyte formation with osteoporotic changes in the later stages.
4. CAT Scan and MRI of spine to access the compression.

Treatment: The treatment available is variable and depends on the stage of spondylosis.

1st stage:

1. Exercises. (as discussed in physiotherapy)
2. Maintain proper posture.
3. Homoeopathic mangement.
4. Cervical traction.

2nd stage:

1. Maintenance of correct posture.
2. Cervical traction
3. Tens and ultrasonic radiations
4. S.W.D. (Short wave diathermy).
5. Homoeopathic management.

3rd stage:

1. Acupuncture is the first treatment of choice.

2. Homoeopathic management.

3. In acute neuropathy, radiation syndrome complete rest and management on traction.

DIAGNOSIS AND INVESTIGATIONS

There are different ways of diagnosing and investigating an arthritic diseases.

Investigations:

1. **Blood examination:** It includes peripheral smear, haemoglobin, R.B.C. Count, Platelets, E.S.R. & R.A. factor complement fixation test. Agglutination tests, uric acid etc.

2. **Urine examination:** Presence of oxalates and urates in the urine are precipitated in case of hyper urecemia.

3. **Radiological investigations:** X-ray and Ultrasound exposures help in diagnosis.

4. **C.T. SCAN:** 5 MRI.

The observation of the physician is the first and foremost requirement to study any disease. The following few observations if noted are useful.

1. **Look of skin:** If dry, parched or oily.

2. **Nails:** White streams, clubbed, psoriatic charges can be seen.

3. **Presence of any nodes:** Could be osler's nodes or hebreden's nodes,

4. Gait of patient how he walks.

5. State of temperature. If the hands are warm it is seen in

RA, thyrotoxicosis even if they are cold then it indicates hypothyroidism.

6.   **Hand shake:** It can be differentiated, as violent handshake of maniac, subdued of melancholic, interrupted of schizophrenic.

7.   **Hand writings:** Inability to write is basically seen in motor agraphia, peripheral nerve lesions.

OBESITY

The ability to store food energy as fat has provided significant survival value to human beings specially in environments where food is either sporadic or scantily available. Because of adequate storage in adipose tissues a normal healthy individual can survive upto 2 months nearly.

Although obesity in itself is a big chapter to choose but it has been deliberately taken here with special reference to "a new concept of body composition analysis (B.C.A.) which is a part and parcel of food and management bureaue. But since it is considered as one of the hindering factors, therefore I have chosen this topic to lay special emphasis on the management of obesity.

Definition and incidence: It can be simply defined as an excess of adipose tissue. But the meaning of excess is hard to understand. Aesthetic considerations aside, clinical diagnosis can be viewed as the degree of excess adiposity that imparts a risk to health. According to "Framingham" 20 % excess over ideal weight imparts health risk. By this way 20 to 30% of men and 30 to 40% of women are obese.

Etiology: When caloric intake exceeds expenditure, the excess calories are stored as fat tissue thus establishing a negative balance.

1. Psycogenic: It is one of the foremost causes of overweight. Persons who are highly anxious and nervous, prone to depressions, mood variations, eat irregularly and often junk foods thus resulting to obesity.

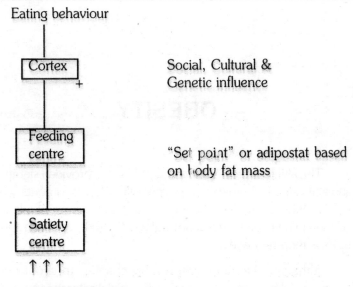

Eating behaviour

Cortex — Social, Cultural & Genetic influence

Feeding centre — "Set point" or adipostat based on body fat mass

Satiety centre

↑ ↑ ↑

1. Gastric distension

2. Plasma Glucose and insulin

3. Adrenergic influences.

2. Secondary obesity

a. **Hypothyroidism.** Obesity results from hypothyroidism due to decreased caloric needs.

b. **Cushing's disease:** It is a rare cause of obesity where typical moonfaces with supraclavicular fat deposits are seen.

c. **Insulinoma:** Hyper insulinemia, secondary to insulinoma ocassionally causes obesity.

d. **Hypothalamic disorders:** Frochlich's syndrome, is primarily presented with obesity. Laurence moon biedle syndrome which is characterised by retinitis pigmentosa, mental deformities, polydactly, syndactly are associated with obesity.

Pathological sequelae of adiposity: It leads to the increased deposits of adipose tissue leading to expanded lean body mass thus causing fatty changes in the visceras leading to impaired functions.

Metabolic sequelae:

1. It leads to hyper insulinemia thus leading to hyperglycaemia.
2. **Diabetes mellitus:** It is the profound effect seen in chronic obese patients.
3. **Hyperlipoproteinemia:** Most plasma cholesterol circulates in the low density lipoprotein and contains most of the triglycerides. Total body cholesterol is increased in obesity.

Manifestations of obesity.

1. Massive obesity induces mechanical physical stress which aggravates or directly precipitates osteoarthrosis and sciatica.
2. Varicose veins.
3. Cholelithiasis
4. Ventral and hiatus hernia.
5. Thrombo embolism.
6. Persistent hypertension.
7. Hypoventillation syndrome: It is also called **Pickwickian syndrome** which leads to apnoea during noctural sleep.

   Body Composition Analysis: It is a highly scientific technique to estimate the exact composition of body which includes:

a. Lean body mass
b. Water content of body
c. Amount of fat.

   Procedure of B.C.A: It is done with the help of a small machine which takes up the feeded data of the patients which includes age, sex, height and weight with related data.

Instructions: 1. It is done preferably empty stomach.

2. During stress or during menses it should be avoided.

3. If the patient suffers from any metabolic disorders then the accepted level of change in the metabolic values should be calculated accordingly.

Steps for B.C.A: 1. Ask the patient to lie down straight on back with hand extended.

2. Apply the electrodes on both the wrist and ankle joints keeping the positive electrode towards heart.

3. Feed all the data and look for all the details on the screen.

Let us look for some cases.

Patient's name	Age	Sex	Height Weight	B.C.A. Total Body
1. Mrs. Urmil Kapoor	43 yrs.	F	165.0 cm 78.0 Kg.	Fat: 48.9% T.B.M: 51.3% T.B.W: 29 Lit B.M.R.: 1363 Cal. T.W.: 25 Kg.
2. Shail Narang	33 yrs	F	152.0 cm 72.0 Kg.	T.B.F.: 43.1 % T.B.M: 56.9% T.B.W.: 30 Lit. B.M.R.: 1385
3. Ms. Neeta Thukral	23yrs	F	157.0 cm 65.0 Kg. 26.5 Kg 30.0 Kg. Target wt. 50.0 Kg.	T.B.F.: 90 % T.B.M.: 60.0% T.B.W.: 28.4 Lit. B.M.R.: 1342
4. Mr. Rajesh	35yrs.	F	173.0cm 97.0 Kg. 63.0 Kg. Target wt: 76.0 Kg.	T.B.F.: 35.1% T.B.M.: 64.9% T.B.W.: 46 Lit. B.M.R.: 1859

5. Puneet Chugh	12 yrs.	M	163.0 cm	T.B.F.: 25.4%
			63.0 Kg.	T.B.M.: 34.6%
			16.0 Kg.	T.B.W.: 74.6 Lit.
			47.0 Kg.	B.M.R.: 1514
			Target wt: 53.0 Kg.	
6. Mr. Sushil Anand	43 yrs.	M	169.0 cm	T.B.F.: 31.6 %
			95.0 Kg.	T.B.M.:68%
			30.0 Kg.	T.B.W.: 47 Lit.
			65.0 Kg.	B.M.R.: 1902
			Target weight: 80.0 Kg.	
7. Mrs. Lata Chugh	30 yrs	F	151.0 cm	T.B.F.: 33.8%
			65.0 Kg.	T.B.M.: 66.2%
			22.0 Kg.	T.B.W.: 31 Lit.
			43.0 Kg.	B.M.R.: 1428
			Target wt: 57.0 kg.	
8. Mrs. Darshana	26 yrs	F	159.0 cm	T.B.F. 32.9%
			70.0 Kg.	T.B.M.: 67.1%
			23.0 Kg.	T.B.W.: 34 Lit.
			47.0 Kg.	B.M.R.: 1514 cal.
			Target wt: 59.0 kg.	
9. Mrs. Aruna Tuli	43yrs	F	148.0 cm	T.B.F. 45.3%
			75.0 Kg.	T.B.M.: 54.7%
			34.0 Kg.	T.B.W.: 29 Lit.
			41.0 Kg.	B.M.R.: 1385.
			Target wt: 58.0 kg.	
10. Mrs. Monika	29 yrs	F	148.0 cm	T.B.F. 46.3%
			80.0 Kg.	T.B.M.: 53.7%
			37.0 Kg.	T.B.W.: 31 Lit.
			43.0 Kg.	B.M.R.: 1514 Cal.
			Target wt: 60.0 Kg.	

Once the readings have been recorded put off the electrodes and wipe off the Gum from the affected parts.

Going through the B.C.A. advice the patient accordingly.

Advantages of B.C.A.

1. It helps in framing the constitutional profile.

2.   It helps in the management of arthritis and all other related disorders.

The clinical aim and importance of B.C.A. is to analyse the human body and predict few problems a head of time.

For eg.: 1. a. If the water retention is more he may have the tendency towards cardiac and renal problems. These problems can be anticipated in near future and helped.

2. If total body mass is more it means the inherent body weight is more therefore foods which cause water retention are to be avoided.

3. It helps to take a balanced and nutritious food.

Note: TB F: Total Body Fats

TBM: Total body Mass

T.B.W.: Total Body water.

B.M.R.: Basal Metabolic rate

Management of obesity: Obesity should not be taken as a symptom but a disease in whole.

1.   **Psycogenic counselling:** Making the patient to understand the importance of balanced, modified but nutritious diet, overcoming stress, improving personal habits.

2.   **Diet modifications:** a. Cut off extra intake of fats, calories. b. Improve roughage in diet. c. Take plenty of water. d. Frame the diet according to your caloric needs rather than physical needs.

3.   **Correction of cause:** If any: If there is any H/o diabetes or any hormonal imbalance, it should be taken care of.

4.   **Physical activity and exercises:** It helps to shed off extra calories and maintain the B.M.R. It can be either brisk walk or a stationary exercise track.

5.   **Nature Cure:** It also helps in reducing and maintaining the

caloric imbalance. This is done with the help of water packs, sand packs and modified regimen. For details look "Naturopathy and nature cure".

6. **Liposuction:** It is a new technique which aims at suction of the extra deposited fats mainly in the hips, upper thighs and buttocks. It is done mainly by two ways.

    a. **Physical/Mechanical Suction:** For this a suction machine attached with a vaccum pump is used. Ask the patient to lie down and a certain amount of vaccum negative pressure is given and sucked with the help of the suction.

    It aims at vaso constriction of local tissues and causing breaking of fats. It is a very painful process and cannot be continued for a long period of time.

    b. **Electro Mechanical Suction:** It aims at breaking the fat deposits by making few linear cuts in this skin. It is done with the help of electrostimulation. By passing mild A.C. current the fat globules are sucked out.

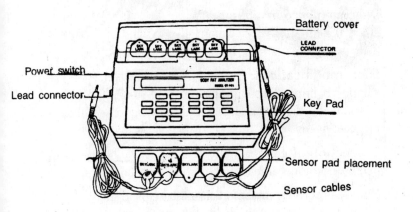

Body Fat Analyser

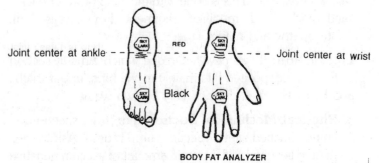

Key pad Sensor pads

Joint center at ankle — — — — — RED — — — — — — — Joint center at wrist

Black

BODY FAT ANALYZER

Liposuction

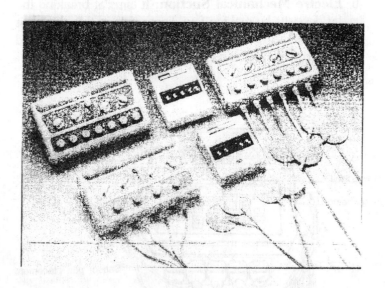

Muscle Stimulator

TREATMENT

Treatment of Arthritis varies from the type of arthritis, it's stages and complications. The type of treatment is decided by the various contributing factors which include the age, general condition and prognosis of disease.

Aim of Treatment: The basic aim of treatment is to

1. Give relief to the patient which includes pain reduction, improving mobility of joint and maintenance of regular physical activities.

2. To reduce muscle spasm, to avoid muscle wasting and to avoid further progress of disease.

3. In a severely affected joint maintenance of case is more important.

There are different modes of treatment which are discussed accordingly.

PHYSIOTHERAPY

Physiotherapy, the so called medicine of physique or physical medicine includes rehabilitation also. According to Bach's "The employment of light, heat, cold, water, electricity, massage, manipulation exercises and mechanical devices .... In the diagnosis and treatment of disease" is scarcely so much a definition as a catalogue of agents which the physical medicine specialist employes; and it omits any reference to the important contribution which the exponent of this branch of medicine makes towards" keeping fit and making the near to fit quite fit be positive health.

Limitation of this recital does not make much sense but a decade back the fusion and integration of special departments took place leading to a special branch of "Physical medicine" the union of these two large tributaries as it were of a - Conference of Technological procedures on one hand and of the wider application of physical training on the other resulted in the river which came to be known as "physical medicine".

Physical medicine plays a major part in the management of the rheumatic patients with the growth of interest in physical medicine, the concept of rehabilitation has acquired a new orientation.

Medical rehabilitation is the process whereby a man is made mentally, physically, socially, vocationally and economically equivalent to his state before he become sick or injured. "It is the fourth leg of medical practice and prevention, diagnosis, treatment and rehabilitation. The physical methods which are applicable to the diagnosis of neuromuscular disorders and peripheral nerve injuries fall into three main groups.

1.   **1st group:** It includes the ways of measuring the nerve and muscle excitability.
2.   **2nd Group:** It records the electrical activity of tissues.
3.   **3rd group:** It tests the integrity of autonomic nervous system (A.N.S.)

The main point in the diagnosis and treatment depends on:

1.   Whether the disease is myogenic or neurogenic.
2.   Level of lesion whether in the C.N.S. Central Nervous System or A.N.S. Autonomic Nervous System.
3.   Lesion is either degenerative or non-degenerative of either sensory or motor origin.

4. Whether any possibility of regeneration is possible or not.

The treatment can be divided in various types depending on the stage of disease.

1. Heat.

2. Massage.

3. Passive movements.

4. Active movements.

5. Electro therapy.

6. Splints and appliances.

7. Occupational therapy.

HEAT

This has been one of the commonest modes of reducing sufferings, be it for arthritic pains or for any abdominal pains (Colic). Application of heat may even be indicated in the acute stage of arthritis. Heat principally improves and increases the local blood circulation with reflex reduction of muscle spasm.

Heat can be either dry or moist heat which can be either mechanical or electrical (discussed later on) with the following ways and means.

1. **Bakers:** It is one of the commonest modes of applying heat. It is usually a U-shaped, polished, slightly curved box with a roof-like reflector on supporting legs. Under this tunnel like reflector, which covers the part to be treated, there are attached from four to sixteen 60 Watt carbon or tungsten filament light bulbs. Such multiple bulb luminous heaters are also helpful in application for back in either lumbar spondylosis or lumbo sciatica syndrome.

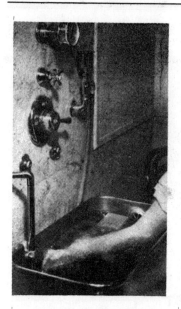
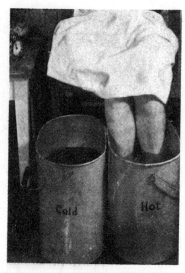
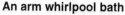

An arm whirlpool bath   **Contrast baths for treatment of lower extremities**

The main advantage of bakers is that in a simple way it can be constructed at home only. The home made baker consists of a curved piece of tin sheet supported on a framework of iron rod. Two double sockets beneath the tin reflector hold four ordinary 60 Watt light bulbs which are connected to the household electric circuit. The specification for the construction of home made baker are as follows: - 17 inches long, 14 inches wide, 14 1/2 inches high over all altitude of arc 5 inches frame. 1/2 inch rod iron, reflector, highly polished, tin sheeting, two porcelain double receptacles; four 60 watt light bulbs. The tin is rolled over the iron rod. The receptacles are connected in multiple with heavy lamp cord, 6 feet long, and a standard plug for connection.

2.   **Lamps for heat application:** It is also useful in applying local heat to the joint. It is a luminous bulb with a cup shaped reflector. The availability of lamp varies from 200 to 1500 watts.

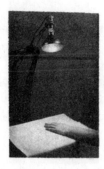

Therapeutic Heating Lamp

Useful:

1. In localised heat to small joints.

2. Less expensive and easy to handle.

3. **Electric Pads:** Pads of light weight containing electric resistance units are occasionally employed for heating joints. The basic advantage of electric pads is it give a uniform heat.

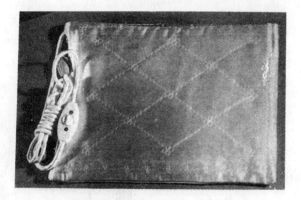

Household Electric Heating Pad

4. **Hot Paraffin packs:** This is one of the commonest and easiest way of heat application. It helps in raising the

temperature of localised parts and can be used without any electrical circuit.

Paraffin wax is melted in a jar, allowed to cool, which forms a thin layer after cooling. The temperature of melting wax should be about 123° to 136° F (50.6°C to 57.8°C). It should be allowed to remain for 20-30 minutes. In cases of rheumatoid Arthritis small joints can be dipped directly in the wax bath or gloves can be worn which can be dipped in the wax bath.

It is useful in

1.   O.A. knees

2.   Rheumatoid arthritis of ankles and smaller joints of hands.

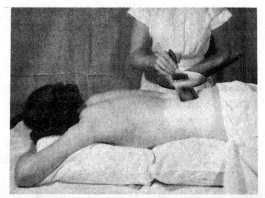

Method of applying paraffin to the back of a patient

Application of a glove of paraffin

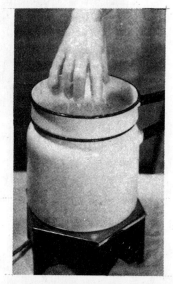

Disadvantages:

1. In few cases allergic reaction of itching, erythema or very rarely blisters may be formed.

2. The method is cumbersome and time consuming.

ULTRAVIOLET RADIATIONS

It is being used as one of the auxiliary measures. In the treatment of rheumatoid arthritis as well as lumbar/cervical spondylosis. It is given with the help of a hot mercury lamp within the sphere of decided dose. Minimal dose is decided by the degree of inflammation. Minimal erythemal dose is given and repeated according to the requirements.

ELECTROTHERAPY

This is one of the commonest modes of physiotherapy which aims at heating of human tissues under a controlled temperature.

The essential Difference between Radiant heating and high frequency heating is the "Depth of penetration. Heating by means of diathermy extends into the deeper tissues of the body. The actual heat depends on the number of calories supplied to the tissues per second by the high frequency current. The heat gradient occurs from without inward. Maximum heat occurring at the point of greatest concentration of the lines of current flow.

There are different modes of heat energy application. It is applied in the form of

a. Long wave diathermy.

b. Short wave diathermy.

c. Microwave diathermy.

1. Short wave diathermy: It is one of the commonest modes which employs: a. The power supply b. Oscillator c. Output or patient's circuit. The high voltage transformer usually has a choke coil in it's primary circuit which controls the output of this device and therefore controls the output of machine.

2. Mercury vapor rectifier tubes: The usual type of mercury vapor rectifier requires 2 ½ volts to light their filaments. The high voltage A-C is fed to the plates of 2-mercury vapor R. Tubes. Each tube passes current during that half of alternating current cycle when the plate is positively charged. With the help of two tubes a pulsating unidirectional current of high voltage is allowed to pass.

For this purpose three different forms of heating techniques are available:

1. **Direct contact heating.** It is a classical method of long wave diathermy where charged metal electrodes are placed in direct contact to the skin or mucus membrane.

2. **Electric or condenser field heating:** The electrodes are separated from the skin or mucus membrane by an insulating layer of air, glass or rubber.

3. **Electro magnetic field heating:** An insulated cable in the form of a coil or loop is coiled around the part or is held against it in a treatment drum

4. **Directional focal method:** It makes use of both the electrostatic and electro-magnetic field. The energy is beamed from an antenna or a radiator and no contact is required for its transmission. This method is employed in short wave diathermy (S.W.D.).

SHORT WAVE DIATHERMY

It is one of the most commonly used modes of heating treatment which is usually available in both small (portable) and a large compact body with A R.F. output upto 250 watts.

It operates at a frequency of 27.1 Hz.

Method of operation:

1. **Illuminated Mains off/on switch:** This switch makes and breaks the main connection to the unit. Set output control to zero before starting on the machine.

2. **Tuning control:** It tunes the output patient circuit of the unit so that it resonates with the final amplifier. This control must always be adjusted to give maximum reading at any selected setting of output power control.

3. **Output control:** This provides the control of output power in 5 steps reaching the patient from zero to maximum position in clockwise direction.

4. **Tuning meter:** This is an indicator for tuning, when the patient's body is properly tuned, switch on the unit, by means of tuning control.

Preparation for treatment:

1. Instruct the patient to remove all metallic objects

   eg.: Pins, Buckles, Coins etc.

2. Clothing should be removed from the area of treatment.

3. Position should always be reclining on table if possible.

4. Comfortable position of patient is very essential for the complete treatment.

Method of using S.W.D.:

1. Apply the 2 electro pads against the opposed surfaces.

2. Always keep a soft cotton cloth between the 2 pads.

3. Switch on the machine, set the output control and the timer (which may vary from 5-10 15-20 min.) depending on the requirement.

4. Heat flow once is uniform, let the patient, be in a comfortable position.

Indications of S.W.D.:

1. Bursitis.
2. Adhesive Capsulitis.
3. Fractures.
4. Osteomyelitis.
5. O.A. and hypertrophic arthritis.
6. Rheumatoid Arthritis.
7. Tenosynovitis.
8. Traumatic injuries.
9. Strains, Sprains and Dislocations.
10. Orifical applications.
11. Gynaecological and Genitourinary conditions.
12. Brachial plexus neuritis.
13. Contusions.
14. Fibrositis.
15. Intercostal rheumatism.
16. Myositis
17. Myalgia.

Contra Indications:

1. It is contraindicated in haemorrhages.
2. Where sensory impairment is marked.
3. In suspected malignancies.
4. In occlusive arterial diseases.
5. In the areas containing metallic implants eg. screws, vitallium cups, plates etc.
6. During pregnancy, low back during menstrual cycle.
7. Application over heart in elderly patients.

ULTRASONIC RADIATIONS

Physical ultrasound solid state is designed to radiate in continuous or pulse form to produce thermal and mechanical effects in the tissues. Ultrasound is capable of separating collagen fibres and of changing the tensile strength of tendons to permit.

Greater extensibility. The mechanical effect have been described as "micromassage" or cellular massage in the deep tissues.

The applicator, transducer a lead zirconate titanate crystal is allowed to radiate ultrasound energy at 1 MHZ with maximum output power of 15 Watts in continuous and 21 Watt peak power in pulse mode. This unit is designed to operate with 230 Volts 50 cycles A.C. power supply.

The operation: All controls and indicators for routine operation of the ultrasonic are located on the top panel. The following are the component parts:

1. **Power Control:** The output power can continuously vary from minimum to maximum and the meter will indicate the output power delivered to the patient.

2. **Timer control:** The timer control switches on the unit. Turn the knob clockwise to set for desired time. Any treatment period upto 15 min will be terminated after the time has elapsed. The switch may be turned off manually or the period may be increased or decreased at will.

3. **Meter:** The meter has two scale S. when the unit is energised power output in Watts per square centimeter is indicated on the lower scale. Total output in watts is indicated on the upper scale.

4. **Ultrasound mode selector switch:** This switch provides selection of continuous or pulsed sound.

5. **Receptor for applicator:** The applicator is to be placed in handle for applicator rest.

6.   **Pilot light:** The pilot light starts to glow when the timer control is turned on and serves to indicate that the unit is energised.

7.   **Output socket:** The applicator male plug is to be connected to the output socket.

Preparation and Operation of the Unit:

1.   Place the applicator on side receptor and power output control at zero.

2.   Attach the applicator male plug to the female socket provided on the front panel and turn clock wise to lock.

3.   Connect mains cable to the unit.

4.   Set ultrasound mode switch for desired mode of operation continuous or pulsed.

5.   Apply liberally mineral or the coupling agent on the area to be treated.

6.   Set pinter of timer control for desired period of treatment. Pilot light should glow immediately.

7.   Unit comes on immediately, ultrasonic power is available at the applicator face.

8.   Remove applicator from the bracket and place it on the area of treatment.

9.   Set power control to desired output as indicated on meter. Start the treatment with sufficient pressure and movement to applicator.

TECHNIQUES OF APPLICATION

Since ultrasonic radiation cannot pass through air, some suitable medium must be provided to conduct the sound from the face of applicator into the tissues. The use of extra mineral oil or a water soluble coupling agent of good efficiency is advisable in a smooth area. In case of an irregular area, or a smaller area, the part should be deeply immersed in water for a better transmission of ultrasonic waves.

1. **Direct application:** In making a direct application, it is essential to use a good film of coupling agent over the entire area to be treated. The applicator is moved with moderate pressure over the skin in a slow and rhythmic manner with a pattern of movement which varies depending on the size and shape of the field to be treated. The movement may be in a stroking manner with the applicator being moved steadily to and fro at a rate of approx four inches per second.

   The applicator may be moved in a circular path at the same rate of the treatment area.

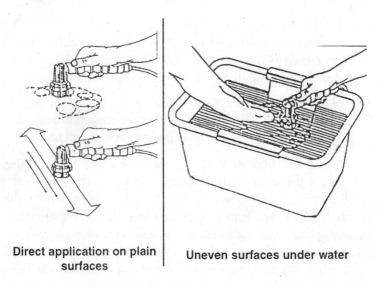

| Direct application on plain surfaces | Uneven surfaces under water |

2. **Spiral way:** In this the applicator is moved in a spiral way over the lapping circles which gives a wide and uniform distribution of waves.

Contraindications:

1. In pregnancy.

2. Sensory impairment.

3. Over the area covering heart, on the head, over the eyes, reproductive organs, directly over the spinal column, directly over the spinal column, visceral plexus and large autonomous gangulia.

   Dosage of ultrasonics: There are various factors which decide and divide the dosage of ultrasonic radiations.

1. Ultrasonic is a safe procedure. Therefore if the dosage is kept below the pain threshold, pain is indication of over dosage.

2. Four to five minutes treatment over the given affected area is sufficient.

3. Therapeutic intensities of 0.5 to 2.0 watts per c.m. have been used with good results. Lower intensities useful in acute conditions while the higher ones in chronic diseases.

4. When ultrasound is applied to the nerve root area, in addition to the affected area the intensity over the nerve root area should not exceed 0-5 watt per square centimeter.

   Ultrasonic dosage is the product of intensity and time. Intensity is the amount of ultrasonic energy being given by the applicator at a given time as indicated by the meter. Time is the duration of the application over any given area. Ultrasound is usually applied with the applicator in motion over the area being treated and it is desirable that the speed of movement be fairly uniform. A rate of approximately 4 inches per second has been suggested as a convenient technique. Following dosage has been suggested for ultrasonic therapy.

Intensity:

1. **Acute cases:** 1 watt per sq. centimeter or less chronic upto 2 watts per sq. cm. time varies from 4-5 minutes.

Few indications for the dosage:

1. Thick tissues such as biceps or buttocks need deeper and prolonged applications.

2. Wider area is covered with increased intensity of ultrasonic radiations.

Combination treatment: Another significant approach is the simultaneous use of electrical stimulation and ultrasound. This application has been useful in the treatment of joint and muscular conditions with sensitive trigger areas. These pain sensitive areas are palpated by means of fingers and both electrical and ultrasonic stimulations are given.

INTERFERENTIAL THERAPY (I.F.T.)

General Introduction: With galvanic and low frequency stimulation it is difficult to get the desired current level through the body due to high skin resistance. Therefore high voltage is given for a better result orientation. When we study the skin physiology, we understand that it can be represented by 100 Ohms resistance. To reduce this impedance one can either increase the value of this capacitance which is rarely possible or the increase the applied frequency. Therefore, by applying a current with a medium frequency, the actual skin resistance is reduced so that once low voltage is required to get the desired current level. on the other hand; for neuro stimulation low frequency vibrations between 0 to 250 Hz are generally used.

I.F.T. gives the combined advantages of both the actions.

Mode of Action: Two oscillators of medium frequency are generated and are cross wisely applied to the body by means of 4 electrode pads. One oscillator has a fixed frequency and 4000 Hz and the other can be between 4000 to 4150 Hz. Both oscillators interfere inside the body, recirculating in modulator signal with 4000 Hz as a carrier and low frequency part for the actual therapy.

With 4 pole I.F.T. two medium alternating current are used which passes through the body with minimum skin resistance and produces a low frequency modulation at the cross over point of the two currents. In this way a specific point in depth of body can be stimulated without much discomfort. The low frequency modulation which exists at the cross over point is utilised only with 2 electrodes.

Using the 2 pole technique, one small electrode is used as a stimulating and searching pad while the other one is used as the neutral pad thus making the process more quicker. A small sweep gradually increasing in range and duration to a total treatment time of 15-20 minutes with a three time toleration dose is given to the tender areas.

Indications of I.F.T.

1. Lumbago (Acute)
2. Osteoarthrosis of knees.
3. Varicose veins.
4. Severe neuralgic pains of A.V.N. (a vascular necrosis of hip joints)
5. Sudeck's Atrophy.
6. Painful Hebreden's Nodes.
7. Intermittent claudication.
8. Capsulitis shoulder with fibrositis.
9. Intercostal neuralgia.
10. Sciatica.

TENS

It is trans electro nerve stimulator. It aims at giving both pulsed and continuous modes of vibrations with the help of an A.C. current.

Principle: The main principle is, it sends electrical impulses through the nerve system thus setting an impulse which reduces the local pain effect.

Method of application: 1. The machine is provided with electrodes and the carbon pads.

2. Ask the patient to show the site of pain.

3. Apply the gel. on the pads and apply pads on opposed surface, tying it with a crepe band.

4. Set the machine according to the requirement and make it either continuous or a pulsed mode. Set it for 15-20 minutes according to the severity of illness.

Utility: 1. Sacro ileitis.

2. Lumbo scral disc prolapse.

3. Lumbago.

4. L.S.S. (Lumbo sciatica syndrome).

5. Varicose veins.

6. Neuropathies.

Complications:

1.Rarely if the patient is anxious and nervous.

2. In neuropathy, burns may develop.

3. Shock symptoms rarely.

TRACTION

It is also one of the modes of physiotherapy which aims at tackling cervical and lumbar spondylosis. It mainly helps in overcoming the cervical spasm by providing a tensile strength to the neck and back as well.

Aim of traction: It mainly aims at reduction of muscle spasm by providing a fixed tensile strength.

It is of 2 types.

1. **Static traction:** It means the tensile strength is made static without any pause which is mainly given in acute sciatica, prolapsed disc.

2. **Intermittent traction:** It means the traction is tensile with an intermittent pause of resting and withdrawl seconds of time.

Indications:

1. Acute cervical spondylosis.

2. Lumbo sciatica syndrome

3. Prolapsed I.V. disc.

4. Acute sacro ileitis.

5. Acute and chronic lumbago.

Method of using:

1. Ask the patient to lie on bed straight with the legs slightly raised.

2. Daignose the patient to calculate the amount of traction to be given.

3. Switch on the machine and start the traction setting on the timer. Allow the patient to rest upon with the pause and free phase of traction.

4. Once the buzzer goes off, machine is automatically switched off.

5. For lumbar traction the lumbar belt of small, medium and large size are used. In case of cervical traction a cervical collar with a tilted rod is used.

Complications:

1. Few nervous patients may get an aggravation response.

2. Very rarely vaso compression may occur leading to diziness or peripheral vasodilatation.

MASSAGE

It is one of the essential steps in the management of arthritis whether rheumatoid or osteoarthrosis although it does not hold much value now. But it helps in improving the blood circulation to the affected joints; thereby reducing the rigidity of joints and thus avoiding contractures.

Contra indications: a. In acute inflammation of joints when heat and redness is marked. b. In contractures. c. In severe pain, massage should be avoided.

Massage not only includes massage but also the movement of affected joints. Direct massage over the joint is avoided, although a mild stroke over the joint helps to alleviate pain.

Indications of Massage:

1. To improve local and general metabolism.

2. To provide a mechanical substitute in aiding circulation for the loss of muscular contractions caused by inactivity.

3. To relieve the pain of myositis.

4. To prevent or delay atrophy of muscle tissue and to assist the restoration of muscle tissue when atrophy has taken place.

5. To improve the blood circulation of the tissues.

EXERCISES

The usual plan for mobilisation of the joint that has been the seat of acute inflammation is to **employ first relaxed (passive) movements.** Later on active assistive exercises in which patient makes an active effort to move the part and is assisted by the therapist in increasing the range of motion are employed.

Finally patient should be encouraged to mobilize the joints by means of active voluntary exercises. Initially these exercises should be practised without weight bearing. Weight bearing should be started only when there is a sufficient range of joint movement to permit moderate extension and flexion of these joints.

Alternate contraction and relaxation of muscle groups and

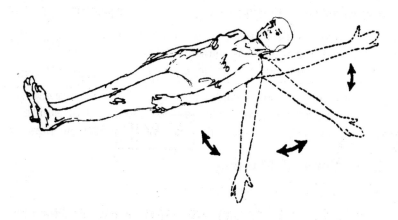

Lie on your back. Raise one arm over your head, keeping your elbow straight. Try to bring your arm close to your ear. Return your arm slowly to your side. Repeat this exercise with your arm. Repeat, alternating arms.

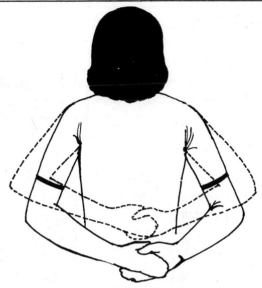

Clasp your hands behind your back. Move your hands up your back to midback. Return down to buttocks and repeat. Remember to keep your head and back erect.

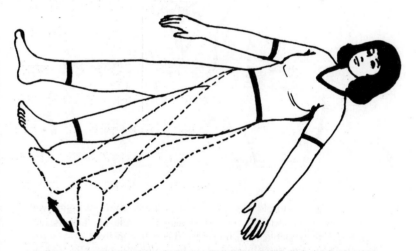

Lie flat on your back with your legs straight and about six inches apart. Slide one leg out to the side and return, at all times keeping the toes pointing straight up towards the ceiling. Repeat, alternating legs.

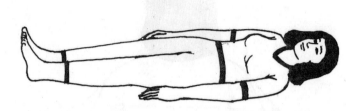

Lie flat on your back with your legs straight and about six inches apart. Roll your knees out, keeping your knees straight. Repeat.

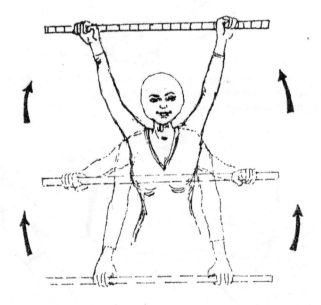

Stand upright and hold a cane or a stick firmly from both ends with your arms extended fully forward. Raise the cane or stick as high overhead as possible. You might try doing this in front of a mirror. You don't have to move both ends to the same height —play around with it. Try rising it to different heights till you reach a comfortable level, then gradually increase your lift.

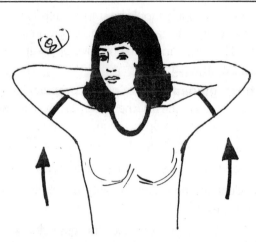

Clasp your hands behind your head. Move your elbows back as far as you can. As you move your elbows back, pull your chin in. Return to starting position and repeat.

their antagonists help in improving the circulation and joint movement aids in maintainance of normal physiological activity.

General Remarks Regarding Exercises

1. When acute inflammation begins to subside this is the first indication for light massage and exercise.

2. The rule of exercise is to avoid any such exercise which may produce pain or precipitate pain.

3. If the joints are more painful the day after exercise then the amount of exercise should be reduced.

4. The morning toilet of arthritic patients shows the beginning of 1st exercise of the day.

5. All exercises should be slow and rhythmic.

6. Jerking motions or pump handle movements should be strictly avoided.

7. Weight bearing should be avoided until it can be tolerated.

8. Knees should always be straightened before walking is

permitted. Walking should be started initially on parallel bars or in a walker. It can be replaced gradually by crutches followed by canes and then objective or unsupported walking should be attained.

9.   **Posture guidance:** To guide properly regarding the posture is also one of the foremost requirements of an arthritic patient. It helps to reduce the trauma to the weight bearing joints and helps to improve the alignment.

Following general rules should always be remembered.

1.   To walk with the weight evenly distributed, feet pointed straight ahead.

2.   Roll the hips under (contract the buttocks downward and abdominal muscles upward). Thereby tilting the pelvis backward and straightening the lumbar portion of spinal column.

3.   Raise the chest upward thereby enlarging the thoracic cavity and raising the diaphragm.

4.   Stretch the back part of the top of head towards the ceiling thus straightening the cervical and thoracic portion of spinal column.

5.   Sit, stand and walk as tall as possible.

SPLINTS AND SUPPORTS

It is one of the most significant part of arthritic management. It helps to avoid contractures and thus giving a complete osteo aid to the disabled.

Common problems which need care are adduction of shoulders, fixation of thorax, kyphosis of thorax, flexion of elbows with special reference to wrists and knees.

The patient with R.A. should lie on a bed that does not sac. In a day he should be allowed to lie without pillows and with all joints extended. Night splints which hold an extremity in extension are useful in preventing potential flexion deformities.

Placing a small pillow under the thoracic part of spinal column helps in hyperextension of spinal column. Padded coil up splints which hold the wrist in dorsiflexion help in avoiding the flexion deformity.

Use of sand bags, pillow or a small splints are useful in presenting or controlling the contractions.

Rehabilitation: Means preparation of the patient physically, mentally, socially and vocationally for the fullest possible life compatible with his abilities and disabilities.

A brief summary of joint exercises is given which helps one to a great extent.

1. Exercises for the upper part of back:

a. Lie down on back; place a rolled bath towel or a small pillow length wise between shoulder blades, place fingers on back of neck, pull arms back, raise chest and return to original position.

b. Lie down on back, place a rolled bath towel or small pillow lengthwise between shoulder blades, with arms straight at the side of body, raise arms upwards, backward over the head as far as possible. Breathe in slowly, bring arms back to original position, breathe out slowly.

c. Lie on abdomen, elbows straight, and arms placed outward from body at right angles, clasp hands behind the back, raise head and chest while straightening elbows forcibly, return to original position.

d. Sit on a chair as straight as possible for count of five to ten with palms of hands at the back of neck, elbows at shoulder level and pulled backwards.

e. Sit with arms folded loosely across the chest, unfold arms, swinging extended arms outward and backward at shoulder level, return to original position.

EXERCISES FOR LOWER PART OF BACK

1. Lying on the back, with legs up on a stool, a folded towel between the shoulders, arms at the sides, hold position for five minutes.

2. Lying on back, draw both knees towards chest, grasp knees with hands and pull them towards chest.

3. Lying on back, draw both knees to chest, roll forward and up to a sitting position.

4. Stand against wall, heels 4 inches from wall, head, shoulders and hips touching the wall, pull in abdomen a push the lower back against wall.

5. Stand 4 inches away from wall, bend body forward at the hips until back is arched, slowly straighten up until the lower part of the back, shoulders and head touch the wall.

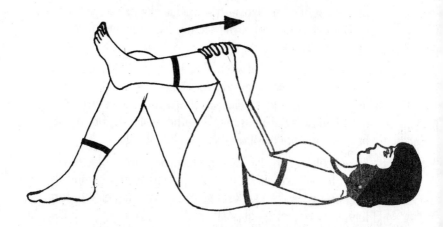

Lie on your back. Bend your knees. Keep your feet flat. Bring your knee towards your chest. Gently bend the knee with your hands and try to touch your heel to your buttock. Do this exercise, one leg at a time.

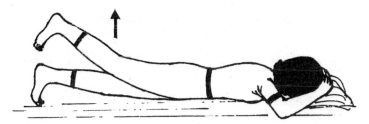

This exercise helps to increase the backward motion of the hip. Lie face down. This alone may provide a good stretch for those who spend a great deal of time sitting or in bed. If this position is comfortable, raise your leg as high as possible. This exercise should not be done by people with low back or disc problems.

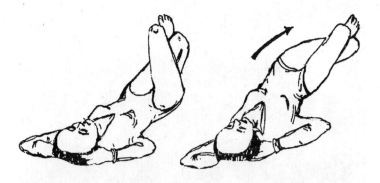

a. Lie on your back, hands out to the side or behind your head. Bend your hip and knees and place feet flat. Cross your right leg over the left knee. b. Rotate hips to the right, trying to touch the knee to the floor. Keep your upper body flat on the floor. Repeat to the other side.

Benefits: This exercise increases the ability of the hip to rotate (roll in and out). This is important for activities such as dancing or rolling over and getting out of bed. This is also a good exercise for stretching the low and middle back, but some may find it too strenuous for the back.

SHOULDER EXERCISES

1. Shoulder struggling in an upward, downward and circular motion.

2. Creeping up the side of a wall with fingers, reaching higher each day.

3.   Arm swinging forward and upward, downward and backward.

4.   Standing fingers interlaced behind the back, turn palms in and out.

5.   Standing arms hanging, wrists crossed in front of body, move arms upwards and backward over head, then return.

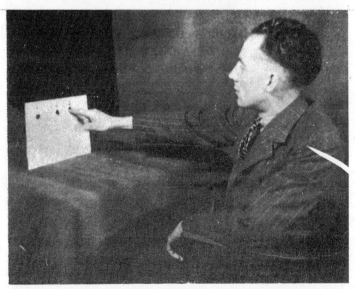

Frenkel's exercises to improve co-ordination of joints of the upper limbs.

ELBOW EXERCISES

1.   Hand touching the shoulder of same side and return.

2.   Pulling up on a bar.

3.   Weight lifting and carrying. Games may be played to increase motion as; throwing a ball, bean bags quoits and sawing wood.

4.   Bending forward over a table, elbow bent palm down on table, palm up on table.

5.   Grasp bar shoulder high, bend knees and exert a pull on elbow.

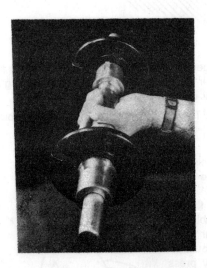

Therapeutic exercises using iron weights-upper extremity.

WRIST EXERCISES

1. Close all fingers and thumb to a tight fist and open to full extension.

2. Standing, facing a table, rest hand palm down on table, hold other hand firmly on top of affected hand, raise elbow and forearm of affected arm slowly upward.

3. Turn a door handle.

4. Wrist shaking.

5. Fingers of both hands bent and grasped by fingers of other hand. Pull gently at first, gradually increase the pull.

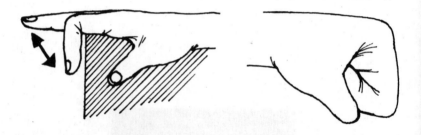

Starting with fingertips, bend each finger joint as much as possible while keeping the other straight. Then make a fist by bending all the knuckles. Open the fist by uncurling the fingers.

Make a tight fist. Then open your hand wide as if grasping a large beach ball. Repeat.

This is an exercise for straightening the joints of the fingers. Place your hand as flat as possible on a table and then place your other hand across your fingers and gently press down, straightening the fingers.

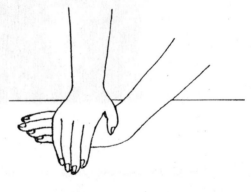

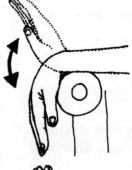

With the forearm resting firmly on a tabletop and the hand hanging over the edge of the table, bend your wrist up as far as possible. Hold. Bend your wrist down as far as possible. Hold. Repeat.

a. Place your hands together by joining the palms and keeping the fingers straight.   b. Press the right hand backward with the left hand, then reverse and press the left hand backward with the right hand. Exert pressure, at the palm and not on the fingertips. Bend the wrist just as possible.

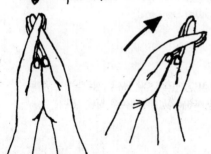

Exercises for Fingers

1. Palm, flat on the table, raise and lower fingers one by one.
2. Make "O" by touching thumb to finger tips one at a time.
3. Crumple a small rubber ball or sponge.
4. Pick up coins; Buttons of assorted sizes.
5. Keep time to music with each finger.

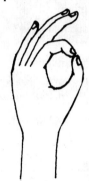 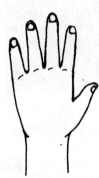

Try to form a letter "O" with each finger and thumb. a. Touch the tip of the thumb to the tip of the index finger, then b. spread your fingers as wide as possible. Proceed on to touch the tip of the thumb to the tips of your other fingers, spreading the fingers wide after each attempt. If you cannot quite bring the thumb to touch the finger, use the other hand to help them bring together gently.

Hip exercises

1. Lie on back, raise and lower leg slowly, with knee straight, with knee bent.
2. Lie on back with legs straight, slide legs wide apart to the side; return.
3. Lie on Back with legs flat on table, stretch first one leg, then the other downward, then shrug hip upward.
4. Go up and down steps.
5. Lie on face and lift leg backward, keeping knee straight.

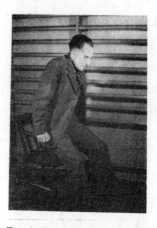

Frenkel's exercises. Patient rising from seated position.

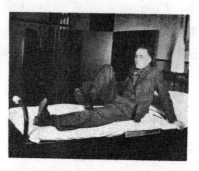

Frenkel's exercises for lower limbs.

KNEE EXERCISES

1. Sitting or lying on back, contract muscles of entire leg, straightening of knee.

2. Sitting leg straight, lift knee off ground.

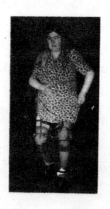

The patient whose knees are X-rayed above shows range of active movement and ability to walk unassisted.

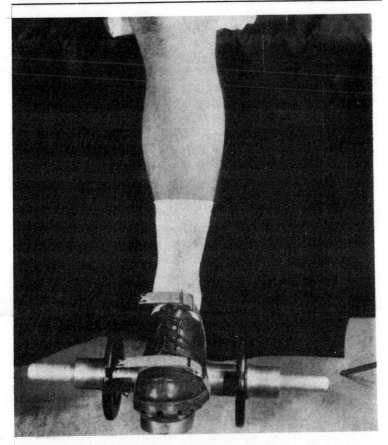

Therapeutic exercises using iron weights-lower extremity.
(Note rolled towel beneath the knee.)

3. Sitting, body errect, legs extended with knees straight, reach forward and touch toes.

4. Lying on back, bicycle legs. Someone grasp feet and give assistance; try to force flexion.

5. Sitting at stall bars, feet against lower rung with knees bent, grasp low bar with both hands and pull body forward.

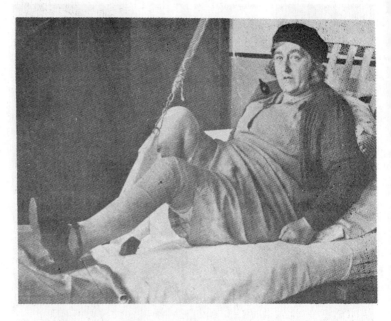

Flexion knee exercise.

ANKLE EXERCISES

1. Alternate bending foot up and down slowly.

2. Alternate turning foot in and out slowly.

3. Sitting, foot circling.

4. Put a bandage or strap across bottom of fore part of foot, hold both ends with your hand, pull up on the bandage, then resist and push foot down, curling toes downward.

5. Sitting, grasp forepart of foot with opposite hand, bending the knee, place hand of same side on knee, push down on knee and pull of on foot, straightening. Let in air.

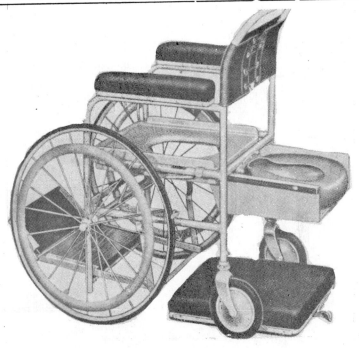

Allwin invalid lavatory chair

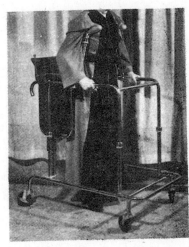

A "walker" which can be employed
for re-education of the arthritic
patient in walking.

Physiotherapy aids rehabilitation in a very smooth way
gradually preparing the patient both physically and mentally.

MAGNET AND IT'S APPLICATION

General Introduction and History

Use of magnets and it's alliances is a new way of treatment specially a drugless way of treatment. The origin of this science dates back to origin of human civilization. Few personalities as paracelsus, andrews etc, had thrown light on it. The oldest mention of magnet as a healing agent is found in atharveda, where in mantras 3 and 4 of sukta 17 of kand 1, of part I speak of the stoppage of bleeding with mantras.

In the 2nd century A.D. Chinese sailors discovered the directive capability of magnets. It was P.A. paracelsus who pioneered work on magnets and brought it to lime light. Dr. William Gilbert of England was the first man to study the effects of electricity and galvinism.

Father Hall, an Australian professor treated nervous men and women by magnet applications.

Use of terminology in magnetism:

The original iron ore which had attracting power and was natural magnet was called magnetic. It was also known as loadstone which means course, journey etc. A magnet is called chumbak in Hindi, Maq natees in Urdu and Persian; Chu shi in Chinese

1. **Magnetism:** A force of interaction between the two magnets and the magnetic material is known as magnetism.

2. **Magnetic pole:** Two small regions, one near each end of

a magnet where the magnetic force is most intense is called "a Pole" respective of the magnet.

3. **North pole and South pole:** When the magnet is suspended freely it sets itself with one pole pointing towards North as north pole and the other towards South, as south pole. North pole Emits blue and south pole emits reddish yellow colours.

4. **Magnetic field:** The space around a magnet in which it's influence is felt.

5. **Line of flux:** It is a line drawn that a tangent to it and any point indicates the direction of magnetic field at that point.

6. **Magnetic flux:** They are the lines of flux in a magnetic field collectively.

7. **Magnetic length:** distance between 2 poles of magnet is magnetic length.

8.. **Magnetic axis:** It is the direction of line drawn from south to north pole.

9. **Magnetic moment:** Of a magnet is the product of it's pole strength and distance between it's poles. It is directed from south to north pole.

10. **Unit pole:** Is one pole which repels an exactly similar pole placed one cm. away in air with a force of one dyne.

11. **Magnetic field intensity:** As a point is the force exerted by the field on a unit, north pole placed at that point.

12. **Oersted:** It is the unit of field intensity. Intensity of field at a point is one oersted if a unit north pole placed there experiences a force of one dyne.

13. **Magnetic induction:** The phenomenon in which pieces of unmagnetised iron or steel are converted into magnets under the influence of a magnet is called induction.

14. **Magnetic meridian:** If a magnet is suspended from it's centre of gravity it point in the north south direction. The

vertical plane passing through it's magnetic axis is called magnetic meridian.

TYPES OF MAGNETS

1. **Natural magnets:** They are those which are naturally found in the form of ores. They are rough and irregular in shape with a weak attractive power.

2. **Artificial magnets:** They are man made magnets which have a strong attractive power. It is prepared by rubbing suitable pieces of iron or any other ferro magnetic substance with a load stone or by passing electric current in a wire coiled suitably around them.

3. **Electromagnets:** They are made by passing a current through a coil wound on a soft iron core. The stronger the current, the better is the resulting magnet. These are temporary magnets which lose their power when electricity is switched off.

4. **Ceramic magnets:** They are the latest research in the development of magnetic field. They are prepared by embedding tiny particles of oxides of Barium and Iron in a ceramic material by the Sintering Process. It gives the highest possible strength.

5. **Bar magnets.**

6. **Cylindrical, solid magnets.**

7. **Ring magnets.**

8. **Chuck magnets.**

9. **Rectangular magnets with and without holes.**

10. **U. shaped/horse shoe magnets.**

11. **Cup shaped magnets.**

12. **Square magnets with or without hole.**

EFFECT OF MAGNETISM ON LIVING LIFE.

Man has been fascinated by the mysterious powers of a magnetic field. The effect of magnetic field is regular and continuous. The constant flow of energy emanating from the magnets cannot be interrupted and it has a continuous influence upon us. We must accept:

1. Magnetically susceptible nutrients such as cobalt, iron, manganese and zinc are although trace elements but play an important role in seedling.

2. A magnetic field can exert without participation of the sense organ, direct effect on diencephalon.

3. Magnetism affects each and every cell of human body.

4. Magnetic treatment has a stabilising effect on the genetic code.

5. It has a strong impact on tissue regeneration, wound healing. Thus helping in tissue fibroplasts regeneration.

EFFECTS OF MAGNETS ON HUMAN METABOLISM

Magnetism is a physical phenomenon which is closely related to electricity also. Magnet has a strong martial attracting power which means any fluid pertaining to iron in the body. In ancient medicine, 4 juices called blood, phlegm, black bile and yellow bile are important.

There are various explanations to have a magnetic effect on the human body.

a. A magnetic field increases the number of crystallisation centres in a liquid which is directly proportional to the strength of magnetic field.

b. When a magnet is brought in contact with the human body. a weak electric current is generated which in turn increases the quantity of ions and thus increasing the ionised blood.

c. It stimulates the hormonal secretions of body thus improving the growth.

d. It regulates the activities of autonomic nervous system.

d. It has a strong eliminative role in excretion of poisonous and waste materials.

g. It helps in energising the self centre of body thus helping to improve the circulation.

APPLICATION OF MAGNETS

Before application of magnets we must understand the polarity of a magnet. Every magnet has a north pole and a south pole. Magnetic lines of force are taken to emerge from the north pole and curl back and converge onto south pole.

The lines of force of a magnetic monopole extends radially in straight lines from the centre of particle likes spokes of wheel. If the line of force extends from the centre it would be a north monopole and if the lines converge towards the centre it would be a south pole.

There are 2 theories which are applicable in application.

a. **Unipolar theory:** It advocates the use of only one pole at a time according to the characteristics of pole.

b. **Bipolar theory:** It is the most widely accepted theory which says "when both the poles are simultaneously applied, they complete the magnetic circuit inside the body which is not achieved by applying a unipolar magnet only.

In general a single pole is used only when the disease is localised. But when generalised the bipolar application is advised.

APPLICATION OF NORTH POLE

1. Arthritis.
2. Bleeding or haemorrhage: After trauma, child birth.
3. Bleeding of wounds, cuts, bruises etc.
4. Boils and carbuncles.
5. Burns.
6. High blood Pressure
7. Sprains in ankles.
8. Any pyogenic infection.
9. Toothache with gingivitis.

APPLICATION OF SOUTH POLE

1. Weak muscles.
2. Neuralgic pains.
3. B.H.P. (Benign hypertrophy of prostate)
4. Improves the internal resistance.
5. In generalised pains, myalgias and myositis.
6. It improves the production of insulin.
7. It improves general blood circulation and hastens the bodily process.

DURATION OF APPLICATION

1. If the disease is in the upper half of body then application is on both the palms.
2. If disease affects lower half of body then under soles of feet is applied.
3. Treatment is given alternately on palms and soles if the disease is generalised.

4. Application is for 15-20 minutes either once or twice in a day depending on the need.

The following are the five ways of magnet application.

Method No.	Pole of Magnet	Where to be applied
I	N.P.	Right hand
	S.P.	Left hand
II	N.P.	Right hand
	S.P.	Left Foot
III	N.P.	Left hand
	S.P.	Left Foot
IV	N.P.	Right hand
	S.P.	Right Foot
V	N.P.	Right Foot
	S.P.	Left Foot

SPECIAL METHODS OF APPLICATION

1. **Eye disorders:** a. Crescent type ceramic magnets are used. N. pole is applied over the closed right eye and S. pole on the left eye for 10 minutes. Eyes are closed for 10-15 minutes. b. South pole of a high power magnet is kept below the (R) palm and N. pole of ceramic magnet on the closed (R) eye then followed by (L) eye.

2. **Ear Disorders:** Apply (N) pole of crescent, ceramic magnet near the outer lobe of right ear on the cheek and S. pole near the outer lobe of left ear on the cheek for 10-12 minutes.

    In the similar way S. pole of a high power magnet may be kept under the (R) palm for 10-12 minutes and N. pole of ceramic

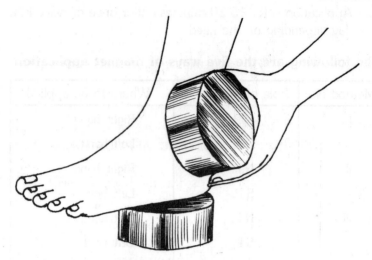

For swollen, stiff and painful ankle: North Pole on the affected ankle and South Pole under the heel.

magnet near the (R) lobe of ear followed by (L) lobe on a dividing time.

3. **For anorectal diseases:** eg: Fissure, haemorrhoids. Both the high power magnets should be kept side by side; N. pole on (R) side and S. pole on (L) side. Patient is asked to sit over it for 15-20 minutes.

4. **For cervical spondylosis:** N. pole to be applied on the affected vertebrae and S. pole towards the radiating side. Treatment is advised early morning for 15-20 minutes.

5. **In knee pains:** N. pole of a high power magnet on the (R) knee and S. pole of magnet on the (L) knee for 15-20 minutes.

GUIDELINES AND GENERAL PRECAUTIONS

1. Take magnet preferably in the morning.
2. Opposite poles of strong flat magnets should not be clapped together.

3. Do not apply magnets immediately after meals.

4. Bath should be avoided at least for 2 hours after application.

5. Do not apply during pregnancy and delicate parts should be avoided.

6. Select the cases suitable for magnetic application.

MEDIUMS OF MAGNETIC APPLICATIONS.

Magnetic rays are accepted in the body in various other indirect forms.

1. **Magnetised water:** Keep a container of water on the bipolar magnet with a iron bar kept between the 2 magnets. It is kept nearly for 24 to 48 hours and is useful in various chronic diseases including chronic amoebiasis, chronic sinusitis. It is consumed gradually once or twice in a day.

Magnetised Water: Water is being Magnetised on both poles. Useful for improving appetite and digestion, helps in reducing constipation and gas formation, also increases urine and drains out stone from Kidneys.

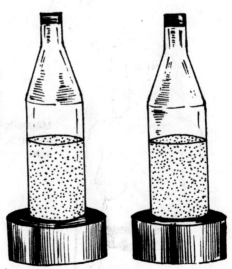

Ovaries: For Pain, Swelling, Dysmenorrhoea and other female disorders including leucorrhoea.

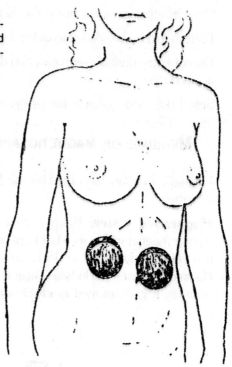

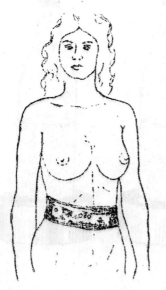

Magnetic Stomach Belt for abdominal ailments, swelling, hernia and backache.

2. **Magnetised Oil:** Method of preparation is similar to magnetic water. It is useful for premature graying of hairs, alopecia, local massage for joints in inflammatory and non inflammatory arthritis.

3. **Magnetic Belts:** Magnets of different strengths wrapped in the form of either knee, ankle, forehead, lumbar belt are used for application.

Let us discuss application of magnets in common ailments

No.	Disease	Method of application
1.	Abscess/Boils	I / V
2.	Acne	I
3.	Adenoids	I
4.	Apthae	I
5.	Asthma	I
6.	Low backache	If horizontal N. pole on (R) and S. pole on (L) side. If vertical, N. pole on upper half, S. pole on the lower portion.
7.	Bronchitis	I
8.	Sinusitis	I with magnetic water
9.	Constipation	II
10.	Seborrhoea	I
11.	Dyspepsia	I
12.	Ear troubles	Discussed in application.
13.	Skin disorders	I or V
14.	Facial palsy	Strong, high power on the affected side.
15.	Fever	I, medium power in the morning and evening. Magnetised water for local compress and oral also.
16.	Gout	I & V.
17.	Hoarseness of voice	I
18.	Insomnia	V
19.	Obesity	I & V
20.	Amenorrhoea	V
21.	P.I.D. (Pelvic Inflammatory Disease)	I & V

ADVANTAGES OF MAGNETOTHERAPY

1. **Time:** It does not consume much time.
2. It is a natural treatment and avoids frequent visits to physician.
3. It accelerates blood circulation and tones up the body in a natural way.
4. It does not have any side effects.
5. It does not require any long preparations.
6. Easy to use, can be handled by anyone.
7. It not only provides treatment and cure but has a prophylactic role also.

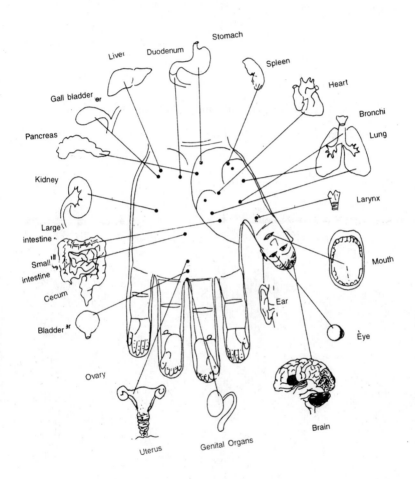

Internal Organs Correspondence Point in Hand

SUJOK ACUPUNCTURE

We have already discussed classical acupuncture in details. Let us study in brief about Sujok Acupuncture. Sujok is a synthesis of different healing techniques based on certain philosophical principles and oriented to relieve human sufferings.

It is a healing method full of spirit which gives it's universal healing power to it's creatures. First publication of Sujok appeared in 1987 when Prof. Park explained it in full details.

Every individual has a metaphysical constitution which cannot be seen but exists and controls all the processes in body thus influencing all the internal organs. A metaphysical constitution is a certain deficiency or excessiveness structure formed by 12 internal organs according to Yin-Yang and five element principles.

The constitution is not a Rigid structure. But only a system of dynamic balance which may change under the impact of certain factors. Disease itself may form a fixed constitution which may be modified by certain factors. In acute diseases, constitution is dynamic and changeable. But in a chronic disease it has a tendency to be fixed with one or several excessive or deficiency factors. In this the metaphysical mode of treatment is given.

The constitution has a tendency to circulate according to the creation cycle of five elements. The distribution of energies may manifest itself at one or the other level; thus giving either a yin or yang constitution.

The first group reflects 3 consecutive excessive bowels as a majority group of excessiveness thus a yang constitution.

Whereas in the 2nd category, 3 consecutive excessive viscera as a majority of excessiveness, giving a Yin constitution. It is named from the central excessive organ of the 3 consecutive viseras or bowels. It can be represented in the human palm. When the fingers are brought together they indicate **excessiveness.** But when they are apart it indicates deficiency.

PRINCIPLES OF SUJOK THERAPY

1. **Six ki:** All the events and objects which are existing can be classified into one of the five element categories. Six ki also corresponds to one of the five elements.

It is a flow of energy which keeps us healthy. When it is well balanced and harmonized we enjoy a sate of health. But on the contrary when it is disturbed disease develops. The six ki are:

1. Wind

2. Heat

3. Hotness

4. Humidity

5. Dryness

6. Coldness.

There is no life on the sun due to imbalanced Six-ki. But heat and wind predominate. Whereas on the earth they have a balance therefore human life exists. Each of Six ki belongs to one of the five elements and interact with each other according to the vital life cycle. With the circulation of seasons, six ki travels through a complex annual change. Every six ki has it's own properties, so let us study it in details.

1. **Wind:** It indicates movements. Every change starts with movement. **Beginning of every phenomenon** belongs

to wind. All the diseases start from wind. In all chronic diseases wind energy is stimulated which regenerates a new life cycle. Spring as a season, with muscle as a body component is important.

Wind subjugates humidity, but is subjugated by dryness. It also antisubjugates dryness. In the six ki cycle wind comes after coldness and creates heat.

2. **Heat:** It follows wind energy in the cycle of circulation. Heat is aggressive in nature and causes warming and expansion. It belongs to 'Fire'. Summer is the season of year with circulatory system as a body component and growth as a part of life cycle.

    When heat is released, movement becomes fast and active and everything grows fast. It is the only factor which works in complete harmony with other six ki. Heat comes after wind and creates hotness yin heat•is supplied by heart Meridian and yang by the small intestine meridian.

3. **Hotness:** It comes after heat in six ki circulation and creates humidity. It is the climax of yang. A point where full growth and ripeness is achieved. When heat is accumulated for a long time, hotness appears. It belongs to maturity.

    Mid summer as the season of year with nervous system as a body component with happiness as emotion, ambition as reason activity and bitter taste belongs to this category.

4. **Humidity:** It dominates primarily during the rainy season. It is the turning point when decline starts. It belongs to "earth" of cycle.

    Late summer flesh as a body component with agony as an emotion is predominant. Itching is one of the most distressful symptoms of humidity.

5. **Dryness:** It dominates during autumn season. It belongs to metal category. Autumn is the season of year with skin and hair as body components. Atrophy is a part of life cycle. With sadness as emotion, pain caused is strong but tolerable.

Yin dryness is supplied by the lung meridian and yang dryness by large intestines meridian.

6. **Coldness:** It predominates during winter. Everything becomes still and warm. Many distressing symptoms as cancer, chronic peptic ulcer etc. belong to coldness.

    Winter as season of the year, with bones as the body components Yin coldness is supplied by kidney meridian. But yang coldness by bladder meridian.

2. **12 types of six ki treatment:** According to six ki constitution a part under structure of deficiency and excessiveness is formed. There are 12 different type of constitutions.

    a. Yang   wind   constitution.
    b. Yin   wind   constitution.
    c. Yin   wind   constitution.
    d. Yin   heat   constitution.
    e. Yang   hotness   constitution.
    f. Yand   humidity   constitution.
    g. Yang   dryness   constitution.
    h. Yin   dryness   constitution.
    i. Yang   coldness   constitution.
    j. Yin   coldness   constitution.

LET US UNDERSTAND CERTAIN POINTS REGARDING
SUJOK:

1. **Correspondence systems in hand and feet:** There are many correspondence system with remote cure and control the functions to prevent and cure the diseases. The hands and feet have a strong resemblance to human body,

therefore it is one of the most important correspondance system.

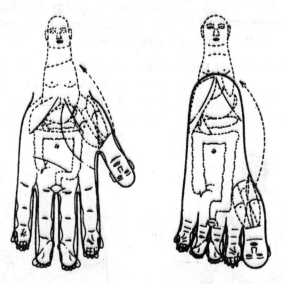

Hand—body correspondence   Foot—body correspondence

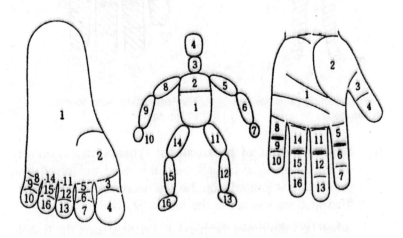

Regional correspondence relation between hand, foot and body

2. **System in hands:** Hands are most similar to human body. The human life exists between the heaven upwards and the earth downwards. This order is reflected in the human body keeping head on the top and reflecting in the thumb, while rest of the fingers pointing towards earth.

3. **Similarity of protrusions:** In the human body there are five protrusions such as the head, left arm, right arm, left and right leg centering around the body: similarly in the hand there are five fingers protruded, centering around the palm.

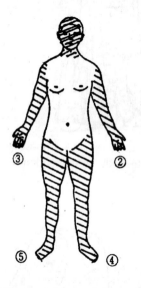

Five projecting parts formed in the body

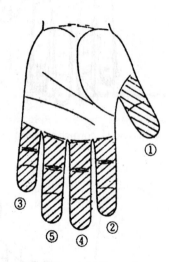

Five projecting parts formed in the hand

4. **Similar height of protrusions:** When a man sits down or stands up in a natural way, the head out of all five protrusions is located atop the two hands are in the middle. Two feet are located in the lowest place.

    When you slip down the hand in a natural way, the thumb is located atop which corresponds to the head. The 2nd and 5th finger located in the middle, which corresponds to two arms, 3rd and 4th fingers are located in the lowest position which correspond to two legs.

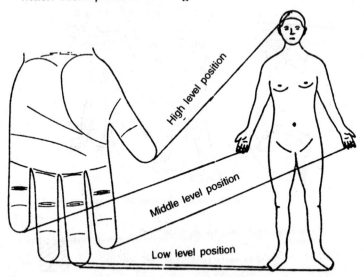

Each of the projecting part in hand and body show the same levels in their natural postures

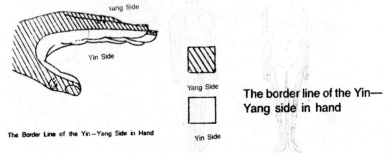

The border line of the Yin—Yang side in hand

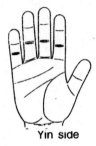
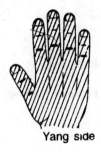

The hand shows clear discrimination between Yin side and Yang side.

Yin side   Yang side

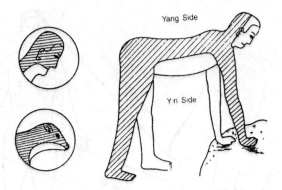

Yang Side

Yin Side

The Body Posture to distinguish Yin side and **Yang** side

(The circles explain native Yin-Yang border ~~line of~~ animal)

line of the human being

Yang Side

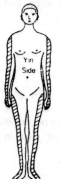

Yin Side

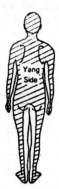

Yang Side

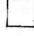

Yin Side

Front side   Back side

Yin side and Yang side of the body

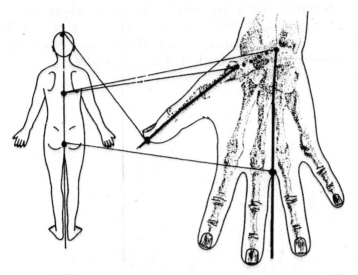

The Yang Center Line of the Body   The Yang Correspondence Center Line of Hand

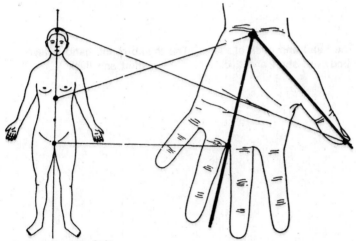

The Yin Center Line of the Body

The Yin Correspondence Center Line of Hand

The comparison of the centre lines in hand and body

5. **Regional parts are similar to each other:** Human body is divided into some parts either by joints and by diaphragm respectively. Similarly hand is also divided into some parts by the borders of hands, knuckles.

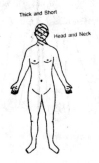

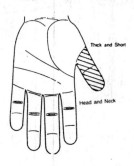

The head and neck of the body are short and thick

The thumb of the hand is also short and thick

Thumb has the central position to control all other fingers

6. **Correspondence in the Yin and Yang area:** Human body is divided into Yin and Yang in the animal position, inside is the Yin area and outer is the Yang. Hand is also divided into Yin and Yang. When clenching the fist, the hiding part of the palm is the Yin area and the exposed part of the back of hand is the Yang.

7. **The centreline corresponds to each other in a symmetry:** The corresponding centreline is the unique centre line which makes perfect symmetry in the anatomic bone structue and number of bones of the hand.

8. **Thumb is the head:** It corresponds to the head out of the five fingers.

   a. It is located on the exact centreline, and located atcp in a natural posture.

   b. **Head has different running directions.** It runs towards heaven and the 2 arms and legs run towards the ground. Head contains the brain which plays a metaphysical role in commanding.

   Protrusion of head consists of head and neck. In the human body, head is divided into two parts such as head and neck and the arms and legs are divided into 3 parts. These three parts are bordered by the wrist, elbow and shoulder joint in the arm, by the ankle joint, knee joint and hip joints in the leg.

   d. **Head controls the arms and legs:** It commands so located in the centre of the arms and legs.

   e. **Head is short and thick:** Head is the shortest and thickest. In the hand too, thumb is short but thicker than the other fingers.

9. **Main correspondence and secondary correspondence:** There are two correspondence points. Main correspondence is an area where exists in the (L) correspondence part of left hand or foot to the left of the

human body, when dividing the body into left and the right with a centreline.

Secondary correspondence is an area where exists in the left correspondence part of (R) hand or foot to the left of human body when body is divided into left and right with a centreline border.

10. **Partial correspondence system:** It is an independent correspondence cure system which covers the roles, the original correspondence structure can't fully undertake and contributes to the preservation of human health.

11. **Correspondence electric wave principles:** The hands feet and the body brings correspondence reaction by electric waves. Similarly when a disease starts it also emits the electric waves. The two types counteract and control the disease process.

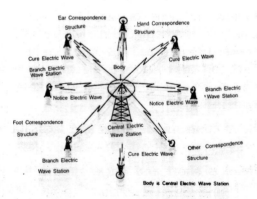

Electronic Wave correspondence relations between the body and the individual correspondence structure

12. **Four axis reflection principle:** In the human body there are four axis and all phenomenon of the body are reflected by the axis to various spots. The metaphysical axis disperse, harmonise the flow of energy thus healing in nature.

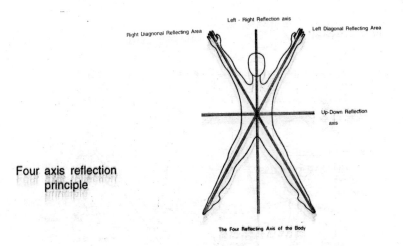

Four axis reflection principle

The Four Reflecting Axis of the Body

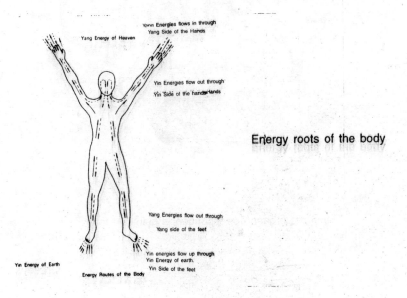

Energy roots of the body

Energy Routes of the Body

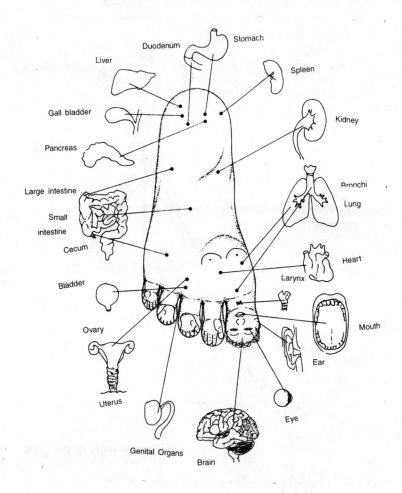

Internal organs correspondence points in foot

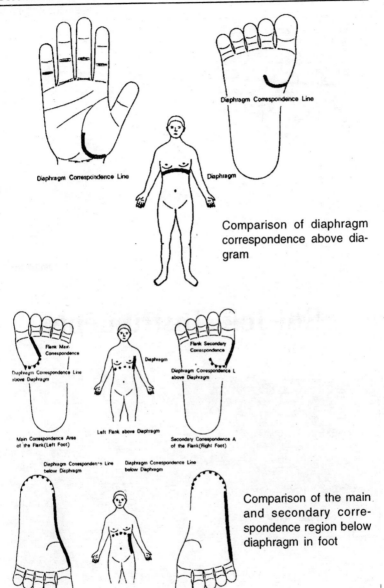

Diaphragm Correspondence Line

Diaphragm Correspondence Line

Diaphragm

Comparison of diaphragm correspondence above diagram

Flank Main Correspondence

Flank Secondary Correspondence

Diaphragm Correspondence Line above Diaphragm

Diaphragm

Diaphragm Correspondence L above Diaphragm

Left Flank above Diaphragm

Main Correspondence Area of the Flank (Left Foot)

Secondary Correspondence A of the Flank (Right Foot)

Diaphragm Correspondence Line below Diaphragm

Diaphragm Correspondence Line below Diaphragm

Comparison of the main and secondary correspondence region below diaphragm in foot

Left Flank below Diaphragm

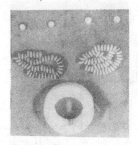

Byol Meridian Magnet

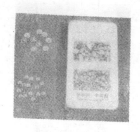

Star Stimulator

Su Jok Instruments

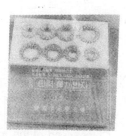

Elastic Ring

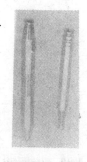

Diagnostic Stick

This is only an introductory study to Su jok. Efforts shall be made to detail the text in the next subject.

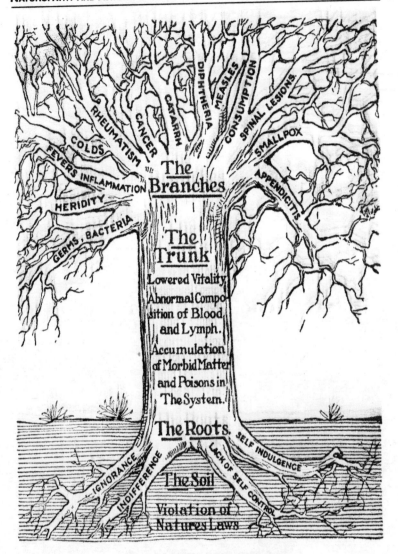

THE UPAS TREE OF DISEASE

Evil is not an accident, not an arbitrary punishment, not always an "error of mortal mind." It is the natural and inevitable result of violation of Nature's laws. It is instructive and corrective in purpose, and will remain with us only as long as we need its salutary lessons.

NATUROPATHY AND NATURE CURE

The Lindkahr system of natural therapeutics represents the first effort ever made to combine in one system, all that is good in various methods of treatment. It is therefore, the only true eclectic system of therapeutics in existence. **It takes in all that is true in old school medical theories and practice, as well as all that is valuable in modern drugless healing methods.**

On the basis of a few fundamental natural laws. It brings **order out of chaos,** simplicity and unity, **out of complexity and confusion.** It reduces the multiplicity of medical and drugless theories and healing methods **to a few simple principles and applications.** It represents one of the most far reaching revolutionary movements in the history of mankind - fundamental to all other reforms, individual as well as social.

It searches for causes of disease and for rational treatment on the physical, mental moral, spiritual, psychial and social planes of human beings. It reveals with irrefutable logic that the **causes of disease and the effects of natural and unnatural treatment are identical** in all domains of human life.

One of the pioneers in the nature cure movement summarised the philosophy of health, disease and treatment in the epigram **"health is cleanliness",** orthodox medicine has learned that this is true as far as surroundings are concerned, but has not yet applied this principal to **internal conditions,** which is proved by the fact that instead of purifying human bodies of morbid waste, systematic poisons and disease taints. It saturates them with drug poisons and disease products, under the guise of medicines, vaccines, serums and antitoxins.

Natural therapeutics or the science of natural healing, does not deny the existence of disease germs and parasites. But claims and proves.

Beyond the possibility of doubt, that these germs and their seed spores, or microzyma, grow and multiply only in bodies heavily encumbered with and weakened by food, drink and drug poisons, morbid taints and various disease products. In the form of vaccines, serums and antitoxins. **In like manner, the drugless healer purifies the human body by** natural methods of living and of treatment, by adjusting mechanical lesions and harmonizing mental and emotional control.

Prof Bechamp, A contemporary of pasteur and metchnikoff, taught as long as sixty years ago that normal cells of living bodies as well as bacteria and other disease producing micro organisms were not the smallest living bodies. But that they were made up of infinitely more minute ferment bodies. He proved that **these microzyma are the principal units of life, which under congenial conditions, develop into normal cells of living bodies.** But which under abnormal conditions, **as in dead bodies, or in accumulations of morbid materials in living bodies,** may develop into bacteria and parasites, whose natural function is to consume and decompose putrefying materials into their component elements. In nature cure it can be expressed as **"every disease germ lives on it's own particular kind of disease matter, and if it does not find this it has to leave for pasteur's new"** or it is eaten by **it's own microzyma.**

Before understanding the concept of disease, we must understand the philosophy of life and health and its application to disease, treatment and cure.

What is life: There are 2 concepts of life material and the vital. The former looks upon life or vital force with all its mental physical and psychical phenomenon and manifests in the form of electric, magnetic and physiochemical activities of human beings. From this angle, life is a sort of **spontaneous combustion or as one** scientist expresses it as **"Succession of fermentations" or chemical changes.**

The vital concept of life regards vital force as a **primary force of all forces,** coming from the great "Central force of life. This force permeates, heats and animates the entire created universe is an expression of **divine intelligence and will the "logos" the word of the great creative intelligence.** It is this energy which sets in motion the whirls in the ether, the electric corpuscles that make up the atoms and elements of matter. It is this **supreme intelligence and power acting in and through every atom, molecule and cell in** human body which is the true healer **"the yis medicatrix naturae"** which always endeavours to repair, to heal and restore the perfect type. All that physician can do is to remove obstructions and to establish normal conditions within and around the patient so that **"the healer within"** can do his work to the best advantage.

After understanding the above details now it becomes easy to understand the placement of health and diseases.

Health: is normal and harmonious vibration of the elements and forces composing the human entity on the physical, mental and moral planes of being, in confirmity with the constructive principle of nature applied to individual life.

Disease: is abnormal or inharmonious vibration of the elements and forces composing the human entity on one or more planes of being in corfirmity with the destructive principle of nature applied to individual life.

To have a better and a positive understanding of the subject we must be in a position to answer few queries which are important.

1. What is nature cure?

Nature cure is a system of man building in harmony with the constructive principle in nature on the physical, mental and moral planes of being.

2. What is the constructive principle in nature?

A principle which builds up, improves and repairs, which makes a perfect individual, and which is opposed to the destructive principle in nature, and whose activity in nature is designated as evolutionary.

3. What is the destructive principle in nature?

A principle which disintegrates and destroys the existing forms and types and whose activity in nature is designated as devolutionary.

4. What is normal or natural?

One which enjoys a harmonic relation with the life principle is natural.

5. What is health?

Health is normal and harmonious vibration of the elements and forces composing the human entity on the physical, mental and moral planes of being, in confirmity with the constructive principle in nature applied to individual life.

6. What is disease?

Disease is abnormal or inharmonious vibration of the elements and forces composing the human entity on one or more planes of being, in confirmity with the destructive principle in nature applied to individual life.

7. What is the primary cause of disease?

Violation of nature's laws barring accidental or surgical causes is the main cause of disease.

8. What are the effects of violation of natures laws on physical human organism?

Following are the effects of violation

a. Lowered vitality b. Abnormal composition of blood and lymph. c. Accumulation of waste matter, morbid materials and poisons.

These conditions are identical with disease, because they tend to lower, hinder or reduce normal body functions leading to destruction of living tissues.

9. What is acute disease?

Acute disease is actually a nature's efforts to eliminate from the organism waste materials, foreign matters and poisons, and to repair the injured tissues. Every acute disease is a cleansing and healing effort of nature.

10. What is a chronic disease?

It is a condition in which the lowered vitality of organism due to accumulation of waste materials and poisons has progressed on, leading to the destruction of vital organs and tissues leading to poor resistance of body.

It is the natural consequence of the inability of the organism to react by acute efforts or "healing crisis" against conditions inimical to health.

11. What is a healing crisis?

Healing crisis is an acute reaction, resulting from the ascendancy or nature's healing forces over disease conditions. It leads to recovery therefore it is a constructive principle of nature.

12. Are all acute reactions healing crisis?

No.

13. What is disease crisis?

It is an acute reaction resulting from the ascendancy of

disease conditions over the healing forces of healing organism. It's tendency is therefore towards fatal termination.

14. What is cure?

Cure is the readjustment of human organism from abnormal to normal conditions and functions.

15. What methods are in confirmity with the constructive principle in nature?

The methods which:

a. Establish the normal surroundings and natural habits of life in accordance with nature's laws.

b. Economize the vital force.

c. Build up the blood on a natural basis with the right proportion of it's natural constituents.

d. Promote the elimination of waste materials and poisons without injuring the human body.

e. Corrects the mechanical lesions.

f. Arouses the individual in the highest possible degree to the consciousness of personal responsibility.

16. Are medicines in confirmity with the constructive principle in nature?

If the medicine is non injurious or non destructive and goes well with the vital phenomenon of body then it is acceptable.

17. Are poisons drugs and promiscuous surgical procedures in confirmity with the constructive principle in nature?

Poisonous drugs and promiscuous operations are in true sense not in confirmity with the constructive principle in nature because;

a. They suppress acute diseases or reactions, i.e. the cleansing and healing efforts of nature.

b. They in themselves are harmful and destructive.

But keeping in mind the vitality of human organism there are certain obstructive factors which nature cannot overcome on her own. Therefore definitely needs some mechanical procedures or forces to overcome such obstacles.

18. Is metaphysical healing in confirmity with the constructive principle of nature?

Metaphysical systems of healing are in confirmity with the constructive principle so far as:

a. They do not interfere with or suppress nature's healing efforts.

b. They increase the inflow of vital energy (force) into the organism.

c. They teach the law of cause and effect and thus awaken and strengthen the consciousness of personal responsibility.

19. Is nature cure in confirmity with the constructive principle in nature?

Nature cure is definitely in confirmity with the constructive principle.

a. It teaches that the primary cause of weakness and disease is disobedience to the laws of nature.

b. It arouses the individual to study nature's laws and demonstrates the necessity of these laws.

c. It strengthens the consciousness of personal responsibility of the individual for his own status of health, for the hereditary conditions, traits and tendencies of his offspring.

d. It encourages and arouses the personal efforts and self help.

e. It assists nature's cleansing and healing efforts by simple natural means and methods of treatment which are not harmful to human life.

20. What are the natural methods of living and of treatment?

a. **Return to nature:** By the regulation of eating, drinking, breathing, bathing, dressing, working, resting, thinking, moral life, sexual and social activities, establishing them on a normal and natural basis.

b. **Elementary remedies:** Like water, air, light, earth, magnetism, electricity etc.

c. **Chemical remedies:** Such as scientific food selection, combinations, homoeopathic medicines, simple herb extracts and vitochemical remedies.

d. **Mechanical remedies:** Like corrective gymnastics, massage, magnetic treatment, structural adjustment and in cases of accidents, surgical intervention.

e. **Mental and spiritual remedies** like scientific relaxation, normal suggestions, constructive thoughts, prayers and meditation etc.

PRIMARY CAUSE OF DISEASE AND IT'S MANIFESTATIONS

The primary cause of all diseases is the violation of nature's laws. It can be in eating, breathing, thinking, dressing, working, resting. Even in moral and sexual behaviour which results in certain primary and secondary manifestations of disease. The 3 primary **manifestations of disease coincide with the three primary life requirements of** the cell.

According to the biological principle the basics of a human being are **innervation, nutrition and drainage.** By innervation, it means a copious influx of life force and an adequate nerve supply from headquarters in the brain and spinal cord. Therefore anything which obstructs, or interferes the nerve connection, lowers the vitality of the cells and thus reflecting **it in either afferent or efferent nerve impulses.**

2. **Nutrition:** This is the 2nd requirement of cell which necessitates the normal composition of blood, lymph and other fluids of body. Therefore abnormal composition of vital fluids constitutes the 2nd primary manifestation of disease.

3. **Drainage:** Accumulation of waste and morbid matter interferes with the drainage as well as with the cell nutrition.

PRIMARY STAGES OF DISEASES

After understanding the causes, we must know how the disease presents itself. It is normally reflected.

1. **Lowered vitality:** Vital force flows uniformly. In the organism which leads to a positive health. More the flow is uniform, more is the resistance and better is the positive health. It is normally expressed as a principled polarity which means either positive or negative. Disease is nothing but a **disturbed polarity.** Exaggerated positive or negative conditions whether **physical or mental or moral** tends to disease on the respective planes of human beings.

    Lowered vitality means lowered, slower and a coarse vibration resulting in a weaker resistance leading to the accumulation of morbid matter, poisons, disease taints, germs and parasites. This is called a negative condition.

2. **Abnormal composition of blood and lymph:** The cells and tissues get their nourishment from the blood and lymph streams. The nutrition of the cell depends upon the nourishment of the organism. Every disease arising in the human organism from internal causes is accompanied by a **deficiency in blood and tissues of important mineral elements** which is caused by an unbalanced diet.

3. **Accumulation of morbid matter and poisons:** It is the tertiary process which leads to an abnormal accumulation of morbid waste materials thus resulting in the tissue clogging leads to various diseases, giving rise to a negative health condition.

Once we have understood the presentations of disease, we must also know how the immune system works to overcome the damaged vitality thus leading to cure and recovery.

1. **Law of dual effect or law of compensation:** Every law has a principle of action and reaction. The great master expressed the ethical application of the law as: **"Give and it shall be given unto you"**.

On its action depends the preservation of energy. Applied to the physical activity of the body. This law can be expressed as: **Every agent affecting the human organism produces two effects: First a temporary effect, second a long lasting effect. The second long lasting effect is always contrary to the first. Transient Effect.**

For eg. The first and temporary effect of a cold application is to send more blood in the interior; but in order to compensate for the local depression, nature responds by sending greater quantities back to the surface; resulting in increased warmth and better circulation. This law governs all drug actions thus regulating the healing process. The initial temporary, violent effect of poisonous drugs when taken in physiological doses is usually nature's role to overcome and eliminate these substances. The 2nd lasting effect is due to the drug retention in the system and their destructive action on the organism.

2. **Suppression versus elimination:** Violation of nature's laws leads to suppression of acute diseases by drug and knife is an important factor leading to malignancy which is generally overlooked.

The following are the cited examples.

1. Diarrhoea is suppressed by opiates thus leading to paralytic bowels i.e. poor or stopped bowel activities.

2. Gonorrhoeal discharges and syphilitic ulcers are suppressed by local injections thus leading to either gastric or urinary troubles.

3. Suppression of epileptic attacks by bromides.

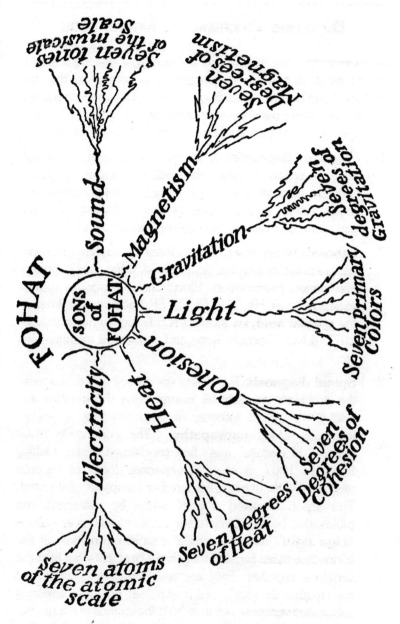

Law of Harmony: Law of Sevens

DIAGNOSIS ACCORDING TO NATURE CURE

Once we have understood the complete disease scale we should be in a position to diagnose our patient so that the treatment can be given accordingly. Careful and complete analysis of each and every patient is very important to conclude the right diagnosis. Following are the steps towards the correct diagnosis.

1. **Physical diagnosis:** It includes a complete thorough analysis which includes the pallor, cyanosis, physique (whether normosthenic, hyper or hyposthenic) clubbing, any pigmentation, scaling or birth marks etc. It also includes the gait, state of muscles, skin colour, mouth odour etc.

2. **Laboratory analysis:** This includes a complete biochemical examination which includes blood, urine, stool, sputum, and semen examination. Blood analysis includes routine examination as, Hb, TLC, DLC, ESR, haemogram. Whereas the **special analysis** includes K.F.T. (kidney function tests) L.F.T. (Liver Function Tests) and serological examinations etc.

3. **Spinal diagnosis:** It is a very specialised way to diagnose the problems specially by manipulating the muscles and testing the spinal integrity. It is checked by a special technique called **naprapathy.** "The connective tissue doctrine of disease" was first proclaimed b Dr. Oakley Smith in 1907. It says "A vertebrae does ot become misplaced without being fractured or completel dislocated. This lesion is called a bony lesion by osteopath and subluxation by the chiropractor but this lesion is actually A **"Liga tight"** which means a shrunken condition of the connective tissue forming the various ligaments that bind the vertebrae together. They are best corrected by means of naprapathic directos". which aims at not only adjusting subluxated vertebrae but stretching the strands of connective tissue. By this technique not only the findings of **tender points** is achieved but they are corrected also by stimulation and stretching.

4. **Irido diagnosis:** It is one of the very important technique to diagnose the diseases are reflected due to improper and altered lymphatic drainage of affected areas.

    Foreg: a. **White streaks** in the iris indicates some gastrointestinal infections or some degenerative changes in the lower alimentary canal.

    b. **Brownish or black streaks** shows an incidental injury to some muscle or a chronic arthritic disorder. Gradually these technique can be learned and practised to get a better diagnosis.

5. **Constitutional diagnosis:** This is also called as face diagnosis. As everybody knows face is the **mirror image of** body which reflects each and everything. In a crude animal, the facial expression is normally a reflection of need may be a desire to eat, drink or to get himself protected from preys. Facial expression is a gift to higher animals of evolution amongst which the human being occupies the first and foremost position. Face not only gives us the external expression but also the internal changes. Therefore it becomes an essential means to diagnose a patient more deeply.

    Facial diagnosis is an in depth attempt to understand the disease and the diseased person but some efforts are made here to make it more clear and perceptible. The facial presentation is normally studied by the area of drainage and its lymphatic channels which is easy to understand.

    Following are the different types of profiles which express and present them as reflecting pictures of internal diseases.

1. Normal average constitution.

    a. Head: Normal.

    b. Forhead: Flat, Mouth a normal layer of fat.

    c. Eyes: Clean, without strain

d. Face: Oval, dividing line clear below the ears.

e. Chest well developed with a normal curved neck.

These type of photographic presentations help us to understand which element in the body is more and which has a tendency to increase or decrease in the ongoing time.

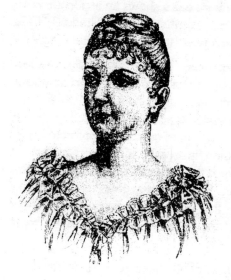

Normal Constitution

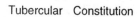
Tubercular Constitution

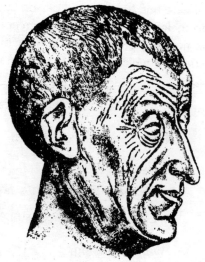

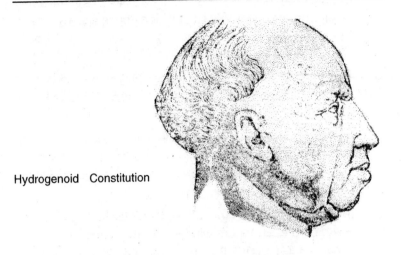

Hydrogenoid   Constitution

TREATMENT AND CURE

Simply identification of sickness is not essential but we must know how to treat a particular disease and whether a problem comes in the scope of nature cure or not. The line of treatment can be studied as

1. General treatment. 2. Specific treatment.

GENERAL REGIMEN / TREATMENT

Here general regimen does not mean the physical cleanliness but an entire change in the system which includes everything as air, water, food clothings, the mental thinking etc. The following indications if followed in a right manner cannot only cure but prevent diseases also.

1. **Mental adjustment:** Mental relaxation is very essential to have a peaceful and good living which helps the patient to self analyze himself. It helps in regulating the inner self with a better control over emotions and higher spirits.

2. **Water sniffing:** It is an excellent way to clear of the nasal

passages thus helps in removing the congestions in the upper respiratory passages. Ideally it is done once early morning. But if repeated 3-4 times in a day is excellent. It helps in chronic catarrhal diseases. It has tonifying effect on C.N.S.

3. **Eye bath:** Eye bathing is done 3-4 times/day and is done with cold water. If eye massage and exercise is done along, gives a dual effect.

4. **Morning drink:** As soon as you get up drink normal tap water around 2-3 glasses if needed one fourth in lemon can also be added. Don't use warm water as it has a weakening effect.

5. **Morning cold rub and air bath:** After bathing exercise nude before an open window. If the temperature and circumstances permit it can be followed by deep breathing exercise and gymnastics. Light exercises with massage also add to the healthy regimen.

6. **Morning walk:** If the weather permits then walking in open air for 15-20 min. is good. If not then punching bag or mild exercises are advisable according to the individual requirement.

7. **Exercises:** It is one of the most important regimen to be followed. It is a splendid form of exercise which helps in elemination of morbid products.

8. **Sun and air baths:** They help in reviving dead skin. It can be taken in combination with regular exercises. Direct exposure to sun rays is not advisable. Air massage is taken either in the morning or at night which helps in releasing both physical and mental strain.

9. **Evening cold sits bath:** It is normally taken with cold water. It should not be taken few days before menstrual cycle. It is beneficial as it draws blood from the periphery and helps in improving the blood circulation.

10. **Eating and drinking:** Good cooking and eating habits are helpful in cultivating a healthy living standard

  a. Do not eat junk foods.

  b. Too much of spicy and oily should be avoided.

  c. One must take ample amount of fruits and vegetables.

  d. Good amount of water should be taken

  e. Fresh, easily digestible food should be consumed.

11. **Frequency of meals:** It is very important to regulate the frequency which gives sufficient time for digestion and assimilation.

12. **Sleep:** Eight hours of sound sleep is the requirement. However it varies from person to person. If needed short afternoon nap can also be taken.

TREATMENT IN ACUTE DISEASES

There are different modes of treatment which are useful in acute disease and are helpful in removing morbid disease products.

1. **Fasting:** Complete abstinence from food is essential in acute febrile conditions. In cases of extreme weakness and acute extreme weakness and acute exacerbation of diseases it is advisable to go for partial fasts which includes giving sort, easily digestible foods as soft boiled egg, buttermilk etc. Once inflammation has entirely subsided then few days should be given to completely heal and repair the broken down tissues. Once fast is broken then small quantities should be given at longer intervals. Following fast patient should be advised to continue on diet with raw fruits and vegetables with good amount of liquids.

2. **Drinking:** As the oxygen demand in febrile diseases is more, so the fluid requirement is also more. But excessive drinking has a weakening effect. Increased production and accumulation of heat leads to more evaporation thereby increasing the requirement of water for elimination of

products through skin, kidneys and bowels. Water should be given freely mixed with lemon juice, grapes and oranges.

a. Flaxseed tea: It is highly recommended for colds, catarrhal diseases and croupy diathesis. It has a soothing and healing effect upon the raw and sore membranes of both respiratory, digestive and urinary organs.

b. Rutabagas: It is also useful in colds and croupy cough, laryngitis etc. It should be taken in a sugar base.

c. Teas: Made from watercress, asparagus or juniper berries have a relaxing effect thus useful in promoting urinary flow in scanty urination.

3. **Hydro therapy:** Use of water as a medicine in a natural way is an old used tradition. But unfortunately it has been applied in a wrong way. The main aim is to:

a. Relieve inner congestion and reflex pain in affected areas.

b. To keep the temperature of affected part below danger point by enhancing heat radiation through skin.

c. To increase the activity of eliminative organs and to facilitate the excretion of waste, morbid products.

d. To increase the positive electro magnetic energies in the system.

e. To increase the amount of oxygen and ozone therapy promoting the oxidation and combustion of waste matter.

Water therapy is usually given in different forms:

1. **Baths and ablutions:** Cold baths are very useful in lowering body temperature. In helps in reduction of inflammation therefore can be used in both antipathic and curative way. If the patient is too weak to get up for bath then cold spray can be used with equal effects. Sprinkle water over the neck, head and body by means of a sprinkler (kneipp cure), bathing spray, pitcher or a dipper. After bath a brisk rub down with a rough towel will help in stimulation

of system. It is one of the most easiest pleasant and refreshing method to treat any kind of fever.

2. **Water packs:** a. whole body pack: It is useful in high fevers where whole body is packed in a wet sheet which helps in inducing sweating. after the removal of pack, a cold sponge is given.

3. **Alternating packs:** If the fever starts taking a strong hold on the body then whole sheet packs are not sufficient to cover up the alternatively packs should be removed only they are warm and given a break in between.

4. **Bed sweat baths:** If the patient does not react to the above packs and remains cold in malaria then sweating is induced with bottles filled with hot water, bricks heated in oven and wrapped, on the lower half of body.

5. **Local compress:** In case of acute inflammation local cold compress can be beneficial. In all fevers with high temperature, it is advisable to keep an extra cooling compress at the nape of neck because thermostatic centres are located here.

6. **Epsom salt treatment:** In severely acute diseases, hydrotherapy is augmented by addition of Epsom salt solution.

7. **Enemas:** It is also one of the beneficial ways in acute diseases. In case of high fever, warm water plain enema is given. But in exceptionally difficult cases injection of warm olive oil is given.

8. **Electro therapy:** During an acute disease lot of energy is required for the increase in oxygen and ozone demands. It is enhanced by passing electric currents through cold packs and ablutions, which help in splitting water molecules into the desired results.

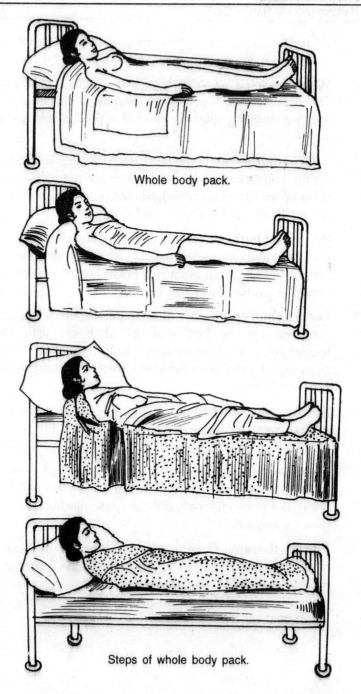

Whole body pack.

Steps of whole body pack.

TREATMENT IN CHRONIC DISEASES
FASTING

One of the most commonest complaints of sick is "Loss of appetite". In majority of cases it is a skill of nature by giving them natural fasting. Loss of appetite is nothing but the overcharged system with excess of pathogenic matter which it tries to get rid of in various forms. Fasting as a remedy is in full harmony with our philosophy of the causes of diseases. Fasting helps in the elimination of morbid waste products. Fasting should be done in a positive way. But once it gives the indications of danger line i.e. appearance of mental depression, psychical symptoms like clairvoyance, sudden loss of weight etc. then it should be checked. It is sage to break the fast before the desired results have been fully obtained and it should be repeated after a period of recuperation. In a disease of chronic origin, preparation of patient is essential by starting low protein. Fat diet rich in positive mineral elements. Raw food diet and through a natural treatment. Therefore, before, during and after a therapeutic fast, everything must be done to keep elimination active, in order to prevent the reabsorption of the toxins that are being stirred up and liberated. There are different kinds of fasts accordingly which can be followed for the particular disease entity.

1. **Regular fast:** In this category, no food is taken. But only sufficient water is taken to quench the thirst. It is a mode to eliminate the morbid waste products.

2. **Dry fast:** It means complete abstinence from water and food as well. It is a difficult way but very useful in highly septic conditions when rapid elimination is necessary. It is advised specially in those people who have obesity or show a tendency for water retention.

3. **Seven day fast:** It is also indicated in diseases of pathogenic origin when the fast is advised for regular 7 days.

4. **The long fast:** These are advocated according to the patient requirement. If need be period can be extended

varying from few days to weeks depending on the need. In between small quantities of acidic fruit juices are added.

But the fast should not be broken abruptly. It needs a proper monitoring specially in regard to the quantity and nature of food taken. Initially the fast should be broken with mild lime juice or a glass of milk or only salted water. It should be followed by gradual intake of salads and fruits and then subsequently light food for few days.

COLD WATER APPLICATIONS

Hydrotherapy has an equivalent effect in chronic diseases which helps in eliminating poisonous morbid pathogenic material in a diseased body. It can be taken in different ways:

1. **Outdoor bathing and swimming:** This activity should never be extended too long. Ideally 20-30 min. is good for it's stimulating effect without any chilliness or exhaustion afterwards. Sea/beach bathing is more beneficial than the ordinary bathing because salt has a positive electromagnetic effect.

2. **Foot bath:** Stand in cold water reaching upto ankles for one or two minutes according to the summer or winter temperature of water. Dry the feet with a coarse towel and rub them vigorously with hands.

3. **Leg bath:** Stand in water upto knees for 2-3 minutes. Rub vigorously to dry and improve the circulation.

4. **Bare foot walk:** On grass or stone pavements is highly beneficial, at least for 15-20 minutes. But if you feel weak then duration can be reduced.

5. **Indoor water treading:** For this standing in a bathtub or large foot tub and splashing vigorously is advisable. To increase the blood circulation. Rub vigorously followed by a mild walk on the floor for few minutes.

6. **Foot spray:** Water is turned with full force from a hydrant towards one foot and followed by other foot. Coldness and force of water will draw blood to the feet. It is useful in improving and normalising the blood circulation. So, helpful in hyperhydrosis of feet: cold, excessive, smelly sweat.

7. **Partial ablutions:** They are useful in local inflammations and congestions thereby helping in localised knee/ankle oedemas and inflammations. "Kalte guss" is an important feature of kniepp cure system. Sprays, showers of short duration is administered at a normal temperature and guss for a short duration.

8. **Limb bath:** Affected limbs are sprayed with water for around 2-3 minutes and followed by brisk rubbing.

9. **Upper body bath:** Stand in an empty tub. Take water in the hollow of hands running from a faucet or a bucket and then rub briskly the upper half of body, from neck to hips for two of three minutes. Use a shower or brush for those Parts which are unapproachable with hands.

10. **Lower body bath:** It is given in the similar way.

11. **Hip bath:** Sit in a large basin or bath tub in enough water to cover the hips completely, legs resting on floor or against the side of tub. While doing the procedure, knead and rub the abdomen, followed by rubbing the skin with a coarse towel.

12. **Morning cold rub:** The essentials for a cold rub are warmth of body before starting, coolness of water, rapidity of action, friction or exercise to stimulate the circulation. It is done by taking the direct heat either from the warmth sitting. In empty bath tub and then followed by gradual cold rubbing with dryness followed from above downwards. This method helps in providing the trio effects of air, exercise, water and magnetic friction of body.

13. **Evening sits bath:** It is taken in a regular tub but if need be an ordinary bath tub can also be used. Water is kept in

the vessel at a level few inches at the natural temperature allowed to fall from the hydrant until a good reaction takes place. Dry with a coarse towel, rub gently and pat the skin with the hands in order to establish a good reaction. It is followed by massage and exercises to get a better effect. This is quite useful in quieting and relaxing the system. It is useful just before going to bed. Cold water draws blood from brain and spinal cord and gives good sleep and rest.

14. **Head bath:** It is useful in seborrnoea and seborrhoeic dermatitis by improving the blood circulation It is taken by dipping small towels in warm/cold water, putting them in groups and covering the scalp with a bigger towel.

WET BANDAGES AND WET PACKS

1. It is a highly beneficial technique in chronic diseases where old muslin, linen sheets, soft towels are used for both bandages and packs. Bandages are used mainly to relief internal congestion, extract heat and to promote the elimination of morbid matter through the skin. Cold water is normally used but if need be then slightly luke warm water may also be used. Bandages are soaked in water, lightly wrung out and applied to the desired body parts.

2. **Wet packs:** It consists of a wet bandage with additional covering of dry flannel or woolen material or of a heavy towel. The dry cover must overlap the upper and lower borders of wet bandage about half of an inch. It helps in exciting and stimulating heat with a warm reaction; thereby preserving the moisture and thus giving a more powerful heating and retaining effect.

The dry cover is normally wrapped in 3-4 layers. The outer end is pinned down and thus helps in retention of heat. **The higher is the fever heat, more vigorous the body heat, thereby wet wrappings more with less dry cover is needed. The lesser is the temperature, low**

is the vitality and reacting heat therefore less wet wrappings and more dry, warm covering is needed.

In chronic diseases, therefore more of dry flannel packing is helpful to provide the lost vital heat.

3. **Vinegar compress and bandages:** It is highly beneficial in **debilitating chronic diseases** where the vitality has been totally shattered. Addition of vinegar and or Epsom salt is recommended. In such compresses quantity may vary depending on the amount of water compress to be used.

4. **Potato compress:** It is applied in local inflammations. In inflamed mucus membranes whereby grated potato is kept in between the flannels and kept for few minutes.

    Ablution after pack: This means the process after the wet pack/bandage has been removed it should be rubbed with a rough towel it helps a. to cleanse the skin of morbid matter. b. It excites a better reaction c. It promotes heat radiation, d. It increases the electromagnetic forces/energies of body.

5. **Whole body pack:** Spread 2-3 blankets on the bed according to the heat; warmth of room and patient's heat. Spread a bed sheet on the blankets which has been wrung out in cold water. Spread a muslin strip over this again wrung in cold water wrap this strip around the trunk then wrap the wet sheet quickly around the body of patient, tucking it in between the legs and also between the body and arms. Pick up the top blanket and took in and around the body, folding the ends in over the feet and around the neck; then pick up the second and third blankets and do the pinning in the same way. Patient begins to react gradually by perspiration and thus feeling comfortable. If he feels too cold then put hot water bottles or bricks heated in the oven with few more blankets if needed let it be for 15-20 min which is followed by a quick but gentle cold rub or a friction rub in bed.

6. **Head bandages:** These bandages are useful in relieving headaches and earaches in order to release the inner

congestion cold pack is used: But since this procedure helps in drawing blood to the affected parts therefore leg/thigh/ throat pack is used to release the congestive headaches. At the same time head, face and neck may be frequently washed or sponged to have it's cooling and refreshing effect.

7. **Throat bandages:** The procedure for application is the same and is specially used in tonsillitis, adenoiditis and chronic pharyngitis.

8. **Throat pack:** It consists of a wet throat bandage plus a covering of dry flannel or wool.

9. **Chest bandage:** It is useful in bronchitis, acute bronchial catarrh and also in pneumonia. Cold wet strip of muslin is tied around the chest from armpits to the border of small ribs and should be wrapped around 3-4 times and removed accordingly.

10. **Chest pack:** It consists of a wet bandage plus a covering of dry flannel or woolen material.

11. **Trunk bandage:** The application procedure is the same as chest bandage but it extends from under the armpits to the upper border of hip bone or pubis. It can be applied in cystitis, appendicitis and oophoritis.

12. **Trunk pack:** It consists of a wet trunk bandage along with a dry flannel or woollen material.

13. **Eye compress:** Wrapped layers of muslin cloth is kept on the eyes and is supported by a dry bandage. It can be accompanied by potato grate. It is highly beneficial in glaucoma, iritis and blepharitis.

14. **Ankle, knee and hand packs:** They are applied to the respective parts in cases of inflammation.

15. **Leg packs:** Method of application is the same. It is highly useful in releasing congestive headaches.

16. **T Pack:** It consists of a narrow strip of muslin adjusted as a belt around the abdomen just above the hip bone to the

back of which is attached a bandage. The wet bandage drawn between the 2 legs. It is useful in high temperatures, inflammations of genito urinary tracts.

17. **Shoulders or scotch pack:** It consists of a packed bandage with flannel which is 6-8 inches wide and one fourth yard long. It is placed around the body under the armpits of the patient, ends crossed in the back and brought up over the shoulders to the front crossing again over the chest. It is useful in chronic and acute bronchitis and bronchial catarrh.

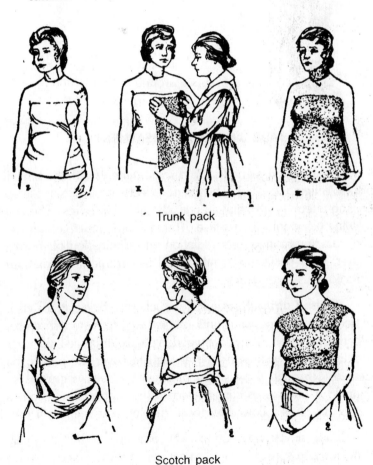

Trunk pack

Scotch pack

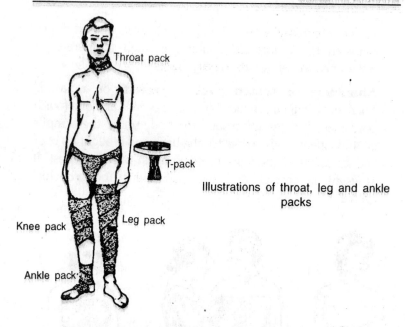

Illustrations of throat, leg and ankle packs

MUD AND CLAY TREATMENT

It is also highly beneficial in chronic ailments with the similar principle being applied. The useful effects are brought due to cooling effect which helps in relaxation of skin pores. Thereby drawing blood into the surface. Thus relieving inner congestion and pain, promoting heat radiation and elimination of morbid matter. Clay packs are highly useful in chronic inflammation, chronic bruises or sprains.

Method of application: Take yellow or blue potter's clay, mascerate in warm water until it is reduced to a smooth paste. When cold spread this with a wooden paddle or broad knife over a strip of cloth wide and long enough to cover the part to be treated. Surround the clay bandage with a few wrappings of flannel or other protecting material. It is kept until it becomes hot or dry. It is followed by towel rubbing and keeping it dry.

In the similar way clay or mud baths are used. In this, clay is heated and spread on a full sheet where it can be covered on the whole body. It is kept for around 20-30 min. followed by warm spray and towel rub with a quick cold spray.

Indications:

1. In chronic rheumatic and arthritic disorders.

2. In chronic gastritis and P.U.S. (Peptic Ulcer Syndrome)

Precautions:

1. Patient should always be explained the procedure.

2. Clay selected should be of a good quality free from dirt, pebbles etc.

3. It is a cumbersome process therefore it should be done in a proper place and under good circumstances.

SUN AND AIR BATHS

Skin is one of the eliminative organs which has both absorptive, assimilative and eliminative properties. This property of skin helps in it's healing effects.

How to take air bath: Whole body is exposed to fresh open air either in the morning or evening according to the temperature. The duration. varies from 10-20 minutes or longer depending on the requirement. It should be a part of regular. Normal routine and is followed by cold rub and exercises.

Sunbath: It is highly recommended in gastric, upper respiratory allergies where whole body is exposed to sun light. The duration may vary from 10-15 minutes initially and can be increased gradually depending on the requirement.

It is of short duration in thin, black skinned people. But can be increased in chubby and fatty people.

Earth magnetism: It is a soothing way of tackling few problems of non pathogenic origin. While taking air bath, if one lies flat on earth or on the back or on belly, then magnetism of earth is absorbed. Walking barefoot has also the electromagnetic reflux from the earth which helps in magnetising and giving a good curative effect. To get in harmony with the great magnetic earth currents, try to lie down with head facing north.

EXERCISES

To keep the body fit one must go for some physical activities which are very essential to keep one healthy both physically and mentally. The first and foremost way to learn exercise is to learn breathing and that too breathing properly.

Process of breathing: We all are aware of the breathing process. In nut shell it is an essential way to life. The effectiveness of breathing exercises depends upon the mental attitude during the time of practise. Putting whole concentration and then taking exercises helps in a better performance.

1.   Always be in fresh and open air, as far as possible.

2.   Take advantage of every opportunity to walk out of doors.

3.   While walking, breathe regularly and deeply filling the lungs to their fullest capacity and also expelling as much air as possible at each exhalation.

4.   Never breathe through mouth.

Method of deep breathing: Following are the steps for a deep breathing exercise.

1.   With hands at sides or on hips, inhale and exhale slowly and deeply, bringing the entire respiratory apparatus into active play.

2.   Expand the chest and increase the air capacity of lungs.

3.   Jerk the shoulders forward in separate several movements, inhaling deeper at each forward jerk. Exhale slowly, bringing the shoulders back to the original position. Reverse the

exercise, jerking the shoulders backward alternating the movements forward and backward helps in completing the cycle of exercise.

4. Stand erect with arms at sides. Inhale slowly, raising the arms forward and upward touching the palms above the head, and raising the toes as high as possible.

   Exhale slowly lowering the heels bringing the hands downward in a wide circle, until the palm touches thighs.

5. Stand errect with hands on hips. In half slowly and deeply raising the shoulders as high as possible.

6. Stand errect, with hands at shoulders. Raising the elbows sideways, inhale gradually. Bringing down the elbows, exhale slowly.

7. Inhale deeply, then exhale slowly. While exhaling clap the chest with palms if hands covering the entire surface.

8. Stand errect with hands on sides. Inhale slowly and deeply, bringing hands, palms up on front of body to the height of shoulders. Exhale at the same time turning the palms downward, bringing the hands down in an outward circle.

9. Stand errect, with (R) arm raised upwards, and left crossed behind the back. Lean far back , bend forward and touch the floor with (R) hand as far as possible without bending the knees. Raise the body to original posture, reverse position or arms and back and repeat the exercise.

10. Errect position with feet well apart, raised arms. Lean back, initially then bend forward, exhaling, touching the floor with both hands between the legs as far back as possible.

11. Horizontal position, supporting the body on palms and toes. Swing the right hand upward and backward, flinging the body to left side, thus resting on the left hand and foot. Return to original position, repeat the exercise, flinging the body to right side. Inhale while swinging backward, exhale while returning to position.

DIAPHRAGMATIC BREATHING

Diaphragmatic breathing is a specialised technique to improve the lung circulation. To stimulate the action of diaphragm lie flat on floor or mattress, the head remains unsupported. Relax the whole body muscles inhale deeply with the diaphragm only. By raising the walls of abdomen just below the ribs without elevating either the chest or the lower abdomen. Take about 4 seconds to inhale, then exhale. In twice by contracting the abdomen below the ribs.

Few general exercises: Have been mentioned which are highly beneficial.

1. Raise the arms forward, upward above the head, and backward, as far as possible, bending back the head and inhaling deeply. Now exhale slowly at the same time lowering arms and head, bending the body downward until the fingers touch the toes. Straighten the knees, inhale again raising arms forward and backward as before. Repeat it 8-10 times.

2. Inhale slowly and deeply with arms at side. Exhale and at the same time bend to the left as far as possible, raising the right arm straight above the head and keeping left arm close to the side of body. Exhale gradually, bending to the right and raising the left arm. **It helps in making the chest flexible. Beneficial in gastritis, gastroenteritis and chronic hyperacidity.**

3. **Chest stretching.** Stand errect and throw the arms back so that the palms touch at the same time, rising on the toes and initialling. Without a pause throw the arms forward and across the chest the right arm uppermost, striking the back, with both hands on opposite sides, exhaling and lowering the toes. Throw the arms back immediately, touching palms, rising on toes and initialing as before, bringing them forward and across the chest again, left arm topmost. It can be repeated 10-15 times.

4. To fill of scrawny necks and hollow chests.

   a. Stand errect without raising or lowering the chin and without bending the neck, push the head forward as far as possible then relax. Repeat it many times. Push the head straight back in similar manner, making an effort to push it farther back each, time.

   b. Stand errect. Bend the head towards right shoulder as far as possible and relaxly repeat the exercise.

   c. Stand errect, bend the head forward as far as possible, making an effort to bring it down further each time. Then bend the head backward.

5. For the muscles of chest and upper arm. Stand straight with elbows to sides. Hands close on chest, thumbs inward. Thrust out the arms vigorously and quickly, 1st straight ahead, then to the sides, straight up and then straight downward. Repeat with up bringing of arms forward and backward from the original position.

6. This exercise helps in stimulating a sluggish liver. Stand errect with hands on hips. Keep the legs straight, rotate trunk upon the hips, bending first forward, then to the right, then backward and then left. Repeat it few times.

7. Lie flat on your back, on a bed or better on the floor with hands under head. Without bending knees, raise right leg as high as possible and lower it slowly. Repeat it number of times, then raise the other leg and alternate. As the abdomen becomes stronger, raise both the legs at once but keeping knees straight. It is important that the legs be lowered slowly.

8. **Stride stand position:** It is highly useful in improving the circulation of genito urinary organs. Stand straight with raised arms on sides until even with the shoulders, without bending the back, rotate the trunk upon hips. First to left and then to right.

9. **See saw motion:** Stand in stride stand position with arms raised sideways. Bend to right until the hand touches the

floor, with high raised left arm. Resume original position and repeat several times.

10. **Chopping exercise:** In stride stand position class the hands above the left shoulder. Swing the arms downward and between the leg, bending well forward. Return to position and repeat number of times.

11. **Cradle rock:** Clasp the hands over head, with elbows straight. Bend the trunk to the right and left side alternately and without pause. Continue for some time.

12. Stand erect with feet together. Jump to the stride stand position at the same time raising arms sideways to shoulders, jump back to original position and lower arms. It can be repeated a number of times.

13. Lie straight on your back with arms at side and legs straight. Raise both legs till they are at right angles with the body. From this position sway legs to right and left alternately.

14. Lie flat on back, with extended arms over head. Swing arms and legs upward simultaneously, touching the toes with hands in midair, balancing on hip bones and lower part of spine it is a difficult exercise therefore should be done carefully.

15. Lie flat on stomach, hands under shoulders, palms downward, with fingers turned inward, about six inches apart. It will give free play to the muscles of chest. Raise upper half of body on hands and arms as high as possible, keeping the body erect and stiff.

16. Lie flat on stomach, arms extended in front. Fling the arms upward and raise the upper part of body as high as possible; keeping legs straight.

17. **Rocking chair motion.** Sit on a mat or bed, legs straight. Arms at side. Recline back so that upper half of body touches the mat, swinging the legs upwards. Return to original position and repeat without pause.

(For pictures refer to treatment chapter)

Special exercises for reducing flesh and strengthening abdominal muscles.

1. Lie flat on stomach, heels and toes together with hands stretched out in front. Fling head and arms upwards at the same time raising the legs with knees kept straight.

2. Similar position with hands clasped on back, feet together.

3. Lie flat on back, hold a soft bar just behind the head. Keep the feet close together and raise the legs as high as possible. Swinging from side to side. Swing legs in a circle without flexing the knees.

4. In the similar position. Raise and lower legs without letting them touch the floor with straight knees.

5. Lie flat on back, fold the hands loosely across the stomach. Raise and lower the upper body without touching the floor.

6. Stand errect with heels together, arms raised above head. Bend forward and downward, endeavouring to place the palms of hands on the floor in front without flexing the knees.

7. Stand errect. raise the arms above the head. Rotate the trunk upon the hips with extended arms, bending as far as possible in each direction, but avoiding undue strain.

GENERAL PRECAUTIONS AND INSTRUCTIONS

1. Do not perform the exercise in high fever, debilitating illnesses.

2. Exercise should not be done on full stomach or immediately after meals.

3. Always learn proper technique and then do exercises.

4. Do not perform heavy, sternous exercises if the body does not permit.

5. Always perform the exercise regularly.

SOLAR THERAPY

It is definitely an old but not very well known branch of natural sciences. It mainly utilises the solar energy for the therapeutic purposes. According to the principle of light, if solar energy is passed through a prism it breaks into 7 visible colours of **vibgyor** i.e. violent, indigo, blue, green, yellow, orange and red. It shows the varying radiations of different wave lengths and refractive index. There is a certain set of rays beyond violet is called as **ultraviolet rays** whereas spectrum beyond red is known as **infrared rays.** Other than these alfa (a) Beta (b), and Gama rays have also been identified. These rays have a strong effect on the human body and they also have a therapeutic effect which is known to have the healing properties.

Every colour has it's own refractive index, mono 7 factor and it's separate wavelength because of which it becomes useful in the therapeutic field. Every colour has it's own property therefore it is used accordingly.

1. **Red:** It has a strong, expanding and irritating effect with resultant heat energy.

2. **Orange:** It is used primarily for the diseases of stomach, spleen, kidneys and intestines. It has a stimulating effect on muscles. It increases the mental power, and improves the mental concentration.

3. **Green:** It has a combined effect of blue and yellow. It is a nature's colour. There it keeps both mind and body active. It also helps in regulating mineral metabolism. It has a stimulating effect and improves the muscle circulation. It also improves blood circulation and acts as a natural therapeutic agent in elimination of pathogenic matters. It is useful in enteritis. Enteric fevers, malaria and chronic fevers; chronic scabies, gastritis and diabetes.

4. **Blue:** It has cooling and soothing effect. It primarily effects throat and upper cervical portion of body. It im-

proves concentration, improves will power. It is useful in high fevers of acute origin. Flu, influenza, hypertension, Insomnia and poor concentration. It can be beneficial in gingivitis, pyorrhoea, diarrhoea, dysentery and food poisoning.

WAYS OF USING SOLAR ENERGY

There are different ways of using sun's rays for it's therapeutic effects. It can be used in following ways:

1. Passing through coloured bottles.

2. Using water as a medium.

3. Air as a medium.

4. Oil as a medium.

5. In a viscous fluid either sugar syrup, milk or honey base. It increases time absorptive power of solar rays.

6. In the latest modes; sand or clay exposed to sun rays is used in debilitating Chronic cases.

WAYS OF USING SOLAR MEDICINES

There are few steps for preparation of these medicines:

1. Take a clean bottle of the same colour (as one needed for the medicine)

2. Fill the bottle with clean water and keep it in sunlight for 6-8 hours. Fill the bottle 3/4 of its volume. Now it is ready to use.

3. Usually medicines of green and blue are given empty stomach or 1/2 hr to 1 hr. before meals. While orange coloured medicines should be given 15-20 min. after meals.

4. The quantity of medicine varies from 3-4 ounces and can

be repeated 2-3 times in the day depending on the requirement.

5. The dosage is decided according to the age of the patient. Dosage is 1 ounce upto 12 years of age and 2 ounces beyond 12 yrs. of age.

6. Similarly medicines in oil or any medium to be used is exposed to sunlight and used accordingly.

7. Every patient has a certain level of element in the body which can be judged by various factors.

   a. Ask the patient to blow air or mirror. After blowing the air takes a specific shape on the mirror. This indicates the excessiveness of that particular element in the body.

   b. Present taste in the mouth will help to identify the gravity of that particular element in the body, thereby it can be used accordingly.

   c. Close the eyes tightly, putting firm pressure and whatever colour appear strongly indicates the deficiency of that colour and thus cán be used as a medicine.

There are certain diseases where it can be used with full confidence.

Name of Disease	Coloured water	Coloured oil/light	Coloured pack
1. All kinds of fevers	Blue or dark blue	Blue light	Blue on navel
2. Dysentery	Blue followed by dark blue		-
3. Arthritis	Orange	On the site of pain: Red followed by blue & followed by deep blue light	Orange strip on Lower abdomen

4. Whooping Cough	Dark blue and orange	- Blue light on head	Blue water gargles - Blue strip on throat.
5. Asthma	Orange, followed by deep blue either separately or combined	- -	-
6.Constipation	Orange	- -	-
7. Gastric flatulence	Orange / deep blue	- -	-
8. Infective hepatitis	Blue or deep blue	- -	-
9. Haemorrhoids	Orange & dark blue followed by dark yellow	- Blue light on the sentinel pile	Blue pack, yellow enema blue water strip on abdomen
10. Boils	-	- Green or blue	Green or sky blue strips.
11. Menopause	Orange 2 times/day	- -	Blue pack on lower abdomen
12. Sinusitis chronic	Orange & deep blue green	- -	Orange & yellow
13. Paralysis	Yellow	- Red for 1 hr followed by blue and all dark blue.	Red cloth followed by exposure to sun
14. Anorexia of psycological reason	Deep blue	- -	-
15. Apthous stomatitis	Blue & Green & yellow	- -	Gargling of green & blue water

The above examples do not give a complete treatment but only guidelines to be followed which helps in choosing the right direction of treatment.

ENEMA AS A FORM OF TREATMENT

General introduction: This is also known as klysmas or colonic flushing and is a simple way of clearing the bowels in a natural way. It is one of the most commonly used steps in the nature cure.

Method of application: The material which is needed for enema is primarily luke warm water available at blood temp between 90°F to 100°F. It is tested by putting a back of elbow in water and noting it down. Poor is the vitality of patient, warmer must be water. In case of subnormal temperature collapse and suspended animation, hot enemas from 100° to 110° F is a powerful tonic. The effect can be improved by adding Epsom salt.

1. Enemas are never taken in the sitting position nor while lying on the right or left side. The ideal way to take enema is to apply knee chest position and lying flat on the back. If the patient is too weak then lying position is advisable.

    a. **Knee chest position:** This posture offers minimum resistance to the passage of warm water through the sigmoid flexure, and the descending and T. colon. Proper care should be taken to dip the hard rubber nozzle of tube into olive oil and tube should not be inserted until the air has been expelled out or water flows from the nozzle at the correct temperature.

Directions to be followed:

1. The entire set of instruments double bag, or can with rubber nose and a flexible rubber tube about 26" long should be kept ready. Rubber tube is fitted to the end of rubber nose by means of a hard rubber connection fill the bag with about two quarts of warm soapy water.

2. Lubricate the colon tube with olive oil. Allow the water to flow until it comes from the Tube at the proper temperature. Stop the flow and insert about 2-3 inches of tube inside the rectum. Release the clip on the nose and allow water to flow.

Gradually push the tube which has been inserted inside.

3. If at the end any irritation or discharge is felt apply over or coconut oil.

Indications: 1. It is indicated in both acute and chronic febrile diseases.

2. In fasting either as a part of fasting or as a part treatment of nature cure.

3. In sluggish bowels specially in diseases of chronic nature.

Contraindications:

1. In severely debilitating illness.

2. In malignancies of lower G.I.T. origin.

3. In pregnancy.

Every system has it's positives and negatives. After going through these details we must know the scope and limitations of every science. Before applying the system one must be aware of the limitations of that system. Nature cure has certain advantages over the other systems in certain ways:

1. Cost effective and economical.

2. Treats without drugs/medicines.

3. Treats in accordance to the laws of nature without violating them.

4. Easy to provide and can be self treated also if within the scope.

5. Gives a cure of the disease.

ACUPUNCTURE AND ACUPRESSURE

General Introduction

Acupuncture is basically one of the most commonly used allied or complimentary system of medicines which started originally in India but was adopted later by Chinese and thus became the inherent adoption of Chinese. Acupuncture is derived from 2 words Acus: needle; punct: to puncture. It is one of the techniques of Chinese system of medicine which originated in the eastern part of China. This art was practised even by the man of stone age when stone needle were used. Eskimos still use sharp stones for treating their diseases. The bantus of South Africa scratch certain areas of skin to treat their diseases. In villages of Saudi Arabia the practise of cauterisation is still quite commonly used. First introductory book on acupuncture was written in Chinese, called **Huang-Di-Nei-Jing** which gives a complete description and conversation between the king Huang di jing and his court physician Chi po.

In traditional Chinese system of medicine, following are the four basic therapeutic methods.

1. **Herbal therapy:** It used the herbs for treatment.

2. **Moxibustion:** It aims at heating or burning few areas of the body with the powdered leaves of moxa plant (Latin word: Artemisia vulgaris)

3. **Acupuncture:** It is in combination with moxibustion used as one of the most ancient and characteristic techniques in Chinese medicine.

4. **Surgery:** This method was used only as a last resort. According to confusion theory, since human body is sacred therefore it should not be traumatised or damaged. It was used only in war injuries and extensive wounds.

Basics and technique: According to the theory of acupuncture, there are 14 channels in our body. There is a continuous flow of energy called Q1 (Prounced as CH1 in Chinese). The energy flows through these channels and it has the same concept as of pran in ayurveda. There are 2 constituents of this energy one +ve called Yang and the other -ve called Yin. In a normal healthy body these two factors are in balance with each other. Whenever there is a deficiency or obstruction in the laminar flow or energy then the person becomes sick with either Yin or Yang energy depletion.

Acupuncture helps in removing this obstructions and thus helps in establishing an equilibrium. There are about 900 points on the whole body surface. Once diagnosis has been made 8-10 points are selected for the treatment and needles are selected according to the sickness or nature of disease. The needles are stimulated with the help of a battery operated machine. The current is of a low voltage and is totally harmless.

Needles are withdrawn after 20-30 minutes. this is known as sitting of acupuncture. This duration may vary from 25 to 30 to 40 minutes also. Needles are removed gently and area is cleaned with a disinfectant.

Theories to explain acupuncture: Acupuncture has now been accepted as one of the most therapeutically useful science which has its sphere and different modes of action. Although certain theories have been brought forward but none gives us a true explanation. The following are certain theoretical explanations.

1. **Neurological theories:** It usually summarises that the perception of pain is modulated by a functional gate within the C.N.S. under normal; conditions. This gate is wide open

and pain impulses get through quite easily. But when needle is applied a second stream of non painful impulses is set up from the site of needling which leads to overcrowding at the gate causing it to close. This results in inhibition of pain impulses and thus no pain is felt.

Under this category few explanation are given which are not discussed in much details.

1. Somato viseral theory: Felix Mann 1960

2. Gate control theory: Melzack and wall (1965).

3. Multiple Gate theory

4. Thalamic integration theory.

5. Thalamic neuron theory.

6. Cortical inhibitory surround theory (Neo pavlovian)

7. Motor gate theory. (Jayasuria and Fernando 1977)

8. Autonomic neuron theory. (Ionescu - Tirgoviste - 1973)

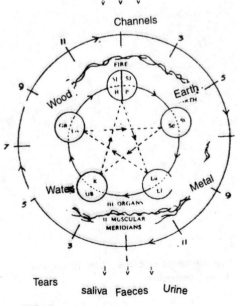

The Three levels of energy
I. Channels.
II. Muscular Meridians.
III. Internal Organs

2. **Humoral theories:** (Neurotransmitter theories)

   1. S. Hydroxytryptamine (Serotomin) : Zhang Xian Gtong.

   2. Endoorphin release theory.

   3. Other neurotransmitters, hormones.

3. **Bioelectric theories:**

   1. Kirlian and Kirlian. (1939)

   2. Becker et al (1976)

4. **Defence mechanism and tissue regeneration theory:**

   Cracuim and others (1973)

5. **Psychological and ideological theory.**

   Theory of hoax or hypnosis (Kroger Et Al 1972.

6. **Placebo effect theory.**

   American medical association (1972)

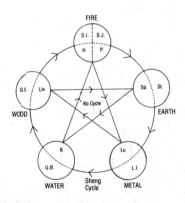

The Relationships of the five elements and the Zang fu organs
Sheng= Generative   Ko= Destructive

7. Catasylophic theory

R. Thom (1975)

8. Traditional Chinese theories of Acupuncture.

Based on Traditional Chinese philosophy.

Effects of Acupuncture: Needless have a multiple sphered seats therefore useful in many conditions. Due to various effects it produces:

1. **Analgesic effect:** It is the physiological basis of Acupuncture anaesthesia and analgesia than others. It is an example of the principle of the specificity of acupuncture points.

2. **Sedative effect:** It causes a reduction activity thus causing sedation. This effect is utilised in the treatment for epilepsy, anxiety, insomnia and neuro and psychological disturbances.

3. **Homoeostatic or regulatory effect:** This is one of the most important activities of acupuncture. It means a homoeostasis between the external and internal environment which is maintained by the balanced activity of sympathetic and parasympathetic and endocrine system.

4. **Immune enhancing effect:** It helps in improving the body resistance due to an increase in leucocytes, antibody formation and gamma globulins

5. **Psychological effect:** It has got a marked tranquilizing action which helps to keep the system calm and cool. It has got a specific action on the mid brain reticular formation and specific brain areas which results in the release of certain chemicals thereby leading to this result.

6. **It improves and hastens motor recovery:** In muscular paralysis. It stimulates anterior horn cells thereby regenerating and reactivating the slow cells thus reviving the slow/dead tissues.

MATERIAL'S USED IN ACUPUNCTURE

I   **Needles:** It is the first and foremost important tool of an acupuncturist. There are several varieties of needles which are used for different purposes.

   a. **Filliform needles:** Every needle has a shaft, head and a tail. The filliform needle has got the similar components but with a long shaft and a filliform tail. The handle may be of silver, copper, bronze, aluminium or of stainless steel. Plastic handled disposable needles are also available. The length of these vary from 0.5 inches to 8 inches or more. The calibre may vary from gauge 26 to 34.

   b. **Embedding needles:** They are thick needles available in different shapes.

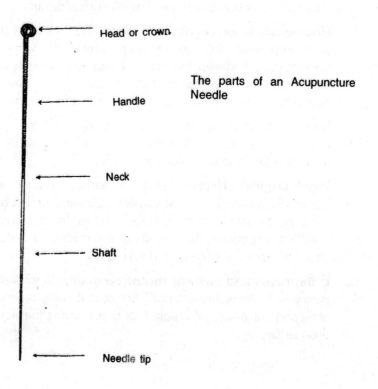

Head or crown

Handle

Neck

Shaft

Needle tip

The parts of an Acupuncture Needle

1. **Thumbtack type:** It appears like a thumbtack with a small circular body in the shape with a diameter of around 3 mm. It is used mainly in ear acupuncture.

2. **Fish tail type:** It is almost similar to thumb talk type except the shaft lies at the similar plane as that of the body. It is inserted horizontally and used in thick tissue areas used for continuous stimulation.

3. **Spherical press needle:** It appears in the ball bearing shape and is used mainly in ear acupuncture. It consists of a tiny stainless steel ball which is fixed on the skin at the site with adhesive tape.

4. **Muscle embedding needle:** It is slightly longer than the fish tail and is used in highly painful conditions like phantom limb or the neuralgic pains of malignancies. To get a better change. It is left in situ at the painful site for few days.

5. **Plum blossom needle:** It is also known as "Five star or seven star" needle. It is made up of 5 or 7 short filliform needles attached to a holder at the end of a long handle. It is used to tap on the skin along a channel or at specific points. It is useful in skin diseases, vitiligo and in those who dislike puncture.

6. **The three edged or prismatic needle:** It is a triangular needle used to bleed certain areas in skin disorders, arthritis and acute emergencies.

7. **The hot needle:** It is a special silver alloy needle which is heated and used to puncture certain superficial lumps like adenomas, ganglions etc.

II. **Electro stimulation:** Normally needles are stimulated manually but when it is done with the help of electrical impulses then it is known as electropuncture. It was 1st invented in China in 1954. It is better than manual stimulation because

    a. It is less tedious, more convenient.

b. It gives a uniform stimulation.

c. It can be done by anybody, without giving much trouble to the patient.

It consists of an electrical apparatus which has got several pulsed modes with a time setter and frequency adjustment control. The frequency variation is selected and the timer is adjusted according to the need may be for 15-20 minutes.

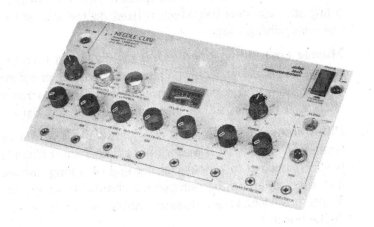

Electro Stimulator and Point Detector

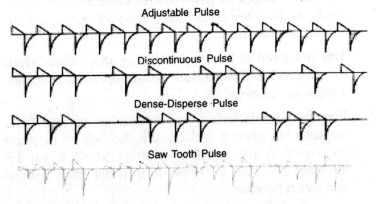

Adjustable Pulse

Discontinuous Pulse

Dense-Disperse ·Pulse

Saw Tooth Pulse

1. Adjustable Pulse   2. Dense-Disperse Pulse
3. Discontinuous Pulse   4. Saw Tooth Pulse

III. **Acupunctoscope:** Acupuncture does not simply mean application of needles but localisation of specific point and then utilising and stimulating these points. The instrument used to detect these points is called an acupunctoscope.

Principle: We all know that the electrical resistance of the skin at an acupuncture point is always less than the resistance in the surrounding area. The point detector helps in identification of these points more precisely. It is used mainly in ear acupuncture.

VI. **Moxa and Moxibustion:** This is one of the sister concern of acupuncture where heating is done with the help of a special herb called moxa "Artemisia vulgaris". It has got special heating properties it is called Zhen-jiu in Chinese it is derived from the Japanese name **Mogusa** for the mogwort plant whose botanical name is Artemisia Vulgaris. Moxa wool is derived by grinding the sun dried leaves of the plant into a fine wool.

STERILIZATION AND DISINFECTION OF NEEDLES

While using the needles the biggest point is the sterilization of needles. The ways of sterilization have been modified gradually with the progress of acupuncture.

Sterilization: Means elimination of all living organisms. Whereas disinfection means the destruction of pathogenic organisms making the object non infective. It may not destroy the microorganisms completely. There are different ways and means of sterilization:

I.   **Physical methods:**

   a. **Heat:** It is the most commonest modes of sterilization. It can be by following means:

1.   **Fire:** A direct flame sterilizes metals at red heat. Needle is held over a spirit lamp flame till the shaft becomes red hot.

2. **Hot air oven:** Hot air is maintained at 160°C for 1 hour or 180°C for 20-30 minutes.

3. **Infrared radiation:** It is used for large scale sterilization. It is maintained at a temperature of 180°C.

4. **Glass bead sterilizer:** It is a mode of dry heat but now used rarely.

5. **Microwave and gamma rays:** Needles are being sterilized by the use of micro and gamma rays.

b. **Moist heat.**

I. **Boiling needless in water:** Boiling needless in water at 100°C for 10-20 minutes destroys most vegetative organisms but few spores may be left.

II. **Autoclaving:** Autoclave is a closed chamber in which objects are subjected to steam at pressures greater than that of atmosphere. Sterilization is quick and time saving.

III. **Radiations:** It is used for plum blossom needles. It is usually a large scale method of sterilization.

IV. **Chemical methods:** It aims at sterilization The help of chemicals. Commonly used chemicals are surgical spirit : 70% alcohol, cetrimide, Chlorohexidine, chloroxylenol etc. This is the most commonest modes of sterilisation.

PRECAUTIONS AND GENERAL INSTRUCTIONS WHILE USING NEEDLES

1. Always make the process clear to the patient and avoid any apprehension regarding the procedure.

2. Always count the needles before and after the procedure.

3. Process should be done gently and calmly.

4. Dangerous or prohibited areas for acupuncture should always be kept in mind.

a. Nipples and breast tissue.

b. Umbilicus.

c. Areas of external genitalia

d. On the wound or burnt area.

There are certain areas which are prohibited for acupuncture:

1. Points of insertion into the orbit of eye: a. $U.B_2$: b. St_6: c. $Ex._4$.

2. Certain points of neck area:

   a. **Front of neck:** Ren_{22}

   b. **Side of neck:** $L_{1\ 18}$ S.I. 17 over the carotid body.

   c. **Back of neck:** DU_{15} over the spinal cord.

   DU_{16} over brain stem.

3. Points over the chest unprotected by bone or cartilage Lu_1, GB_{21}.

4. Liv_3 It can cause overcorrection be causing sudden hypoglycemia in diabetics; too lowering of blood pressure in hypertensives.

5. Points in close proximity to the blood vessels

   Eg. Lu_9, P_3.

6. St_{21}, on the right side as it over lies the gall bladder area.

CONTRA INDICATIONS TO ACUPUNCTURE

There are certain ailments where acupuncture has a limited role therefore it becomes a contraindication for the system.

1. **Cancer and malignancy:** It does not have a curative role but can be used as a palliative mode in secondary manifestation of malignancy for Eg.: Anorexia, severe neuralgic pains, insomnia etc.

2. **Mechanical obstructions:** In absolute mechanical obstructions like twisted loop of intestine, severed tendon etc. It has a limited role.

3. **Surgical indications:** In fractured bones, dislocation, congenital disorders eg. cleft lip, ano cleft palate etc.

4. **Pregnancy:** In the first 3 months and last 3 months of pregnancy it is contraindicated.

5. **Fulminating infections:** It can be combined with drug therapy but only acupuncture alone has a limited role in talking acute infections specially of pyogenic origin.

6. **Patients on multiple medications:** If the patient is overloaded with drugs then the homoeostatic action of acupuncture may cause either hypovolemia, hypoglycemia, hypotension accordingly. Therefore the situation is managed accordingly.

7. **Haemorrhagic diseases:** In diseases like hereditary telengectasias, haemophilia etc. it is contraindicated.

8. Miscellaneous conditions.

   a. Very old and debilitating patients.

   b. Who sweat profusely.

   c. Who suffers from vasovagal shocks.

   d. Immediately after intercourse/hot bath etc.

COMPLICATIONS DUE TO ACUPUNCTURE

Usually no complications have been reported due to acupuncture but certain accidental reportings have been seen most likely due to improper techniques, or lack of skill etc.

1. **Pain:** It is one of the most commonest complaint and can be due to:

   a. Bad acupuncture.

   b. Hypersensitivity of patient.

   c. Bad needles.

   d. Bad posture of patient.

2. **Bleeding:** It is a very mild complaint related to the withdrawl of needles. It is checked by massaging the point with a dry cotton swab

3. **Fainting:** It is commonly seen in nervous and over anxious patients; or due to tiredness, general weakness, hunger etc. It can be avoided by educating the patient, giving him a comfortable posture and understanding him psychologically.

4. **Bent: Broken or stuck needle:** Sometimes the needle is bent or broken. Patient should be restored to his original position and then needle should be handled.

5. **Infection:** Practically it is very rarely seen but sometimes crop up as a problem if the needle is not sterilized properly.

6. **Forgotten needle:** It is a very common error. Therefore needles should always be counted.

7. **Abortion or premature delivery:** If done during 1st and last 3 months of pregnancy it can cause uterine contractions and may lead either to abortion or premature delivery.

8. **Injury to internal vital structures:** It ococures rarely but can be avoided by further precautions carefully.

9. **Electro acupuncture complications:** If the machine is not of a good quality then certain complications may be seen.

   a. Electrocution due to short circuiting or transformer break-down.

   b. Electrical burns: If without needles, electrostimulation is carried out.

   c. Ventricular fibrillation or cardiac arrest may occur.

   d. Interference of cardiac pace makers.

   e. Burns from infra red lasers.

   f. Headache due to over exposure.

ANATOMY OF ACUPUNCTURE

Before needling it is very important to understand the anatomy of acupuncture application. In prehistoric times Chinese discovered that there were certain points of the body which if massaged, punctured or heated have a pain relieving effect. With the passage of time many such points were discovered and it was found that by stimulation of widely separated points it was possible to influence the functioning of specific internal organs. These points were then systematically arranged on the basis of pertaining organs and were connected to form a channel.

Thee are twelve regular channels called twelve paired channels, eight extra channels called **extraordinary** channels. Each of the twelve paired channels relate to one of the twelve internal organs. As the internal organs six channels are Yin and six are yang. The eight extraordinary channels run on the midline one in front (ren channel) and the other in the back (DU). These two channels have their own points. Since only ren and du channels possess their own points therefore they are paired with twelve of the twelve paired channels, six traverse the arm of the six channels serving the arm three are Yin and Run on the anterior aspect of upper limb centrifugally. **The three Yin channels** of hand three are Yang and Run centripetally on the posterior aspect of the upper limb. The three Yang channels of hand. Likewise of the six channels serving the lower limb, three are yin and Run centripetally on the medial aspect of leg. "Three Yin channels of foot" 3 Yang channels Running centrifugally on the anterior, lateral and posterior aspect of lower limb. "The three yang channels of foot the 3 Yin channels of hand commence from the chest and flow to the hand where they meet with the 3 Yang channels of hand near nails. The 3 Yang channels of hand commence from the hand, ascend to the head, where they meet 3 yang channels of four.

The 3 yang channels of foot commence from head, run towards the foot and meet the 3 Yin channels of foot.

The 3 Yin channels of Foot commence from the foot, ascend to the chest and meet the three yin channels of hand.

All organs above the diaphragm are Yin. They are lung, heart and pericardium. They are connected to the 3 Yin channels of hand. All solid organs below the diaphragm are Yin they are spleen, kidney and liver. They are connected to the three yin channels of foot.

Amongst the yang organs, 3 are connected to 3 yang channels of hand. They are large intestine, small intestine and sanjiao (the three body cavities. The other three, Yang are connected to the three yang channels of foot. They are stomach, urinary bladder and gall gladder.

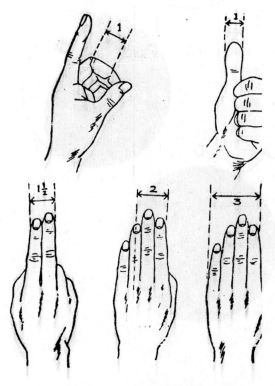

1 cun = 10 fen.
2 cun - 21/2 fin-
ger breadths (of
the patient).
5 cun = 6 1/2 fin-
ger breadths (of
the patient)

Finger Measurements

YIN & YANG

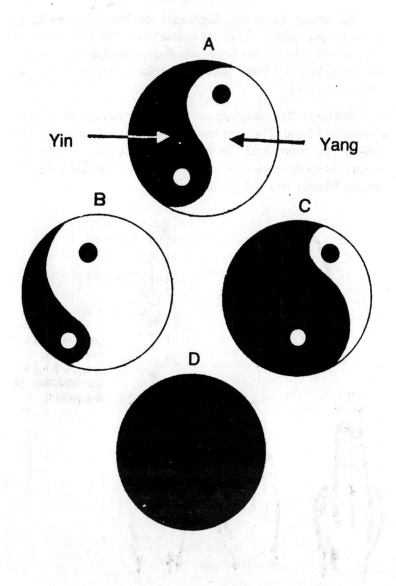

A — Health   B — Excess Yang   C — Excess Yin   D— Death

FIVE ZANG ORGANS

The five zang organs: Store the vital essence of the body they are:

1. **Heart: (H) Pericardium (P):** The Chinese term for this organ refer to both the heart and cerebrum (B). It regulates the blood circulation and improves mental activity. Heart opens to the tongue and governs the blood vessels. It couples with small intestine.

2. **Lung (Lu):** It regulates respiration and opens to the nose. It governs skin and body hair and couples with the large intestine.

3. **Spleen (Sp):** It regulates digestion, controls metabolism of water and also circulatory function of blood. It governs muscles, soft tissues and all 4 limbs. It supplies nutrition to the tongue, and lips opens to the mouth, Coupling with stomach is the main presentation.

4. **Liver (Liv):** It stores and regulates the blood billiary secretion is controlled. It opens to eye and couples with gall bladder.

5. **Kidney (K):** The concept of kidney in traditional Chinese medicine includes the genital functions it regulates bone growth, teeth, cartilages and scalp hairs. It opens to ear and couples with urinary bladder.

SIX FU ORGANS

The Fu organs digest and absorb food and excrete the wastes.

1. **Stomach: (St.):** It regulates ingestion, digestion and transport of food and water.

2. **Small intestine (S.I.):** It separates the essence from waste of food and transports the latter to large intestine.

3. **Large intestine (L.I.):** It is one of the main organs of excretion.

4. **Gall bladder (G.B.):** It controls the mental activities, stores bile and maintains the integrity of muscles.

5. **Urinary bladder (U.B.):** It controls water fluid circulation.

6. **Snajiao (S.J.):** It maintains the homoeostasis of body.

Colours of various structures is very important in making a diagnosis.

1. Colour of mouth (tongue): Heart and pericardium.

2. Colour of Skin: Lungs.

3. Color of lips: Spleen.

4. Color of nails: Liver

5. Colour of Ears: Kidneys.

FEW EXPLAINED PRINCIPLES OF ACUPUNCTURE

1. Organ Clock theory: The energy in this world goes in a cyclic fashion. Similarly energy flows in these 12 channels in a cyclical fashion and is called by the name of organ clock.

3 a.m. - 5 a.m.	Lung.
5 a.m. - 7 a.m.	Large intestines
7 a.m. - 9 a.m.	Stomach
9 a.m. - 11 a.m.	Spleen
11 a.m. - 1 p.m.	Heart
1 p.m. - 3 p.m.	Small intestine
3 p.m. - 5 p.m.	Urinary bladder
5 p.m. - 7 p.m.	Kidney
7 p.m. - 9 p.m.	Pericardium
9 p.m. - 11 p.m.	Triple warmer
11 p.m. - 1 a.m.	Gall bladder
1 a.m. - 3 a.m.	Liver.

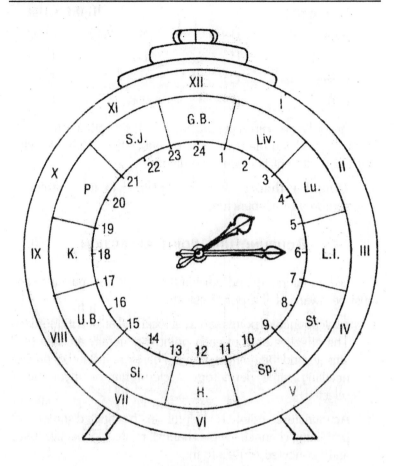

The Organ Clock
Showing cyclical flow of energy

2   **Theory of Yin and yang:** Nature explains two equal and opposite forces eg. sun and moon, woman and man, heat and cold etc. As man is a part of nature, similar principles is applied to the human body.

   Pulse diagnosis: It is carried out with 6 fingers: 3 at each wrist. It can be explained.

Left wrist		**Right wrist**	
Superficial	Deep	Superficial	Deep
S.I.	H.	L.I.	L.U.
G.B.	Liv.	S.I. '	Sp.
U.B.	K.	T.W.	P.

According to some acupuncturists K. is on both wrists instead of 'P'. By studying the pulse, energy imbalance can be detected and the treatment is given accordingly.

4. **Zang Fu theory:** Already explained in the chapter of anatomy of acupuncture.

ACUPUNCTURE POINT SELECTION

Before taking up and starting the case for acupuncture one must be aware of the points selection.

1. All acupuncture points can treat local and adjacent disorders: The effective area of each point is generally an area of 2 cms around the point on limbs. Therefore instead of precise needling same dermatome, sclerotome or myotome is selected.

2. Acupuncture point is helpful in treating disorders of pertaining channel, couple channel, related connective tissue and connected sense organs.

3. Acupuncture point can treat disorders along the pathway of the meridian. Needling on dangerous point can be prevented by taking a remote point on true distal points: The points lying away from the site of action are called distal points. Mostly these points lie below the elbow or knee but treat proximal disorders. They are also known as **remote points.**

The following are the distal points:

1. **Hegu LI$_{14}$:** For diseases of forehead, front of face, front of neck, eye, ear and nose.

2. **Lieque: Lu$_7$:** For the diseases of back of head, neck, and lungs upper half of back.

3. **Neiguan P$_6$:** For diseases of thorax and abdomen.

4. **Zusanli ST$_{36}$:** For abdomen.

5. **Sanyinijao Sp$_6$:** For perineum.

6. **Weizhong UB$_{40}$:** Lower half of back, lumbar region, urogenital disorders etc.

Other few distal points are:

1. **Lanwex Ex $_{33}$:** For appendix.

2. **Dannang Ex $_{35}$:** For liver.

3. **Tiaokon St$_{38}$:** For shoulder.

4. **Houxi S$_{13}$:**   For neck.

5. **Waiguan Tw$_5$:** For temporal headache.

5. **Influential points:** They are specific points.

   a. **UB $_{11}$:** For bone and cartilage (useful in arthritis, spondylosis etc.

   b. **UB $_{17}$:** For blood (Leukemia, anaemia)

3. **Ren $_{12}$:** For hollow organs (P.U.S., indigestion, Constipation etc.)

4. **Ren. $_{17}$:** For lung tissue (Bronchial asthma, bronchitis etc.)

5. **Gibby:**   For muscles and tendons.

6. **GB $_{39}$:** Bone marrow. (Aplastic anaemia)

7. **L.U.$_9$** Blood vessels. arteriosclerosis, varicose veins)

8. **Liv $_{13}$:** For solid organs (Cirrhosis, nephritis, glomerulo nephritis, etc.

6. **XI:** Cleft points: Each channel has a point which is useful in treating the acute disorders of that channel, for eg.

   St 34: For acute pain in abdomen.

K5: For renal colic.

Lu.6: Acute attack of asthma.

These points need strong electrical stimulation for a magic effect.

7. **Yuan source points:** This point has the maximum stored energy in that pertaining channel. It is useful in treating chronic disorders. These points lie close to either wrist or these points lie close to either wrist or ankle. for eg:

1. **Liv$_4$:** For chronic constipation.

2. **Liv$_3$:** For hepatitis.

3. **Lu.9:** For Bronchial asthma.

4. **K3:** Nephritis.

5. **H7:** Heart or brain disorders.

8. **Jingwell points:** They are used in acute emergency. They lie on the ends of channels generally on the toes and fingers except Du26, K.

a. **Du$_{26}$:** In coma, heart attack.

b. **K$_1$:** Snake bite, coma.

c. **H$_9$:** Heart attack.

d. **Lu.$_{11}$:** In respiratory failure.

According to the principle of acupuncture, emergencies are due to excess Qi. in these channels. Thereby, puncturing these points by triangular needle, excess energy is escaped and thus balance of Qi level is achieved.

9. **Ah shi point:** These are the tender points which must be touched and stimulated for a cure.

10. **Alarm point:** This point usually warns about the disease of related channel. It becomes tender if the channel is affected. They are also called mu-front points. They help in diagnosis, treatment as well as the prognosis of diseases.

Most of them lie on ren channel. Alarm points on the back are called **back shu points.** They lie on the medial branch of urinary bladder channel.

11. **Luo connecting points:** This point connects the main channel to it's Yuan source point.

12. Diseases of one side of body can be treated by choosing points of either side, as both halves are connected to each other through ren or du. For eg: In neuralgias, psoriasis, eczema etc. points of opposite side are used.

Let us study each channel in detail so that a complete framework is formed.

LUNG MERIDIAN

It is connected to lung, large intestine nose, skin and body hairs.

1. **Lu.1: Zhongfu.**

Location: (a) At the level of intercostal space between first and second ribs, 6 cun lateral to midline (b) In the infraclavicular fossa 1.5 c.m. below the midpoint of the clavicle.

Indications: a. Cough, pain chest and shoulder area, lung diseases, bronchial asthma etc.

It is the mu front point of lung thereby rendering it tender in lung diseases. Needling is done 0.5 c.m. laterally and horizontally moxa is applicable in chronic bronchial asthma.

2. **Lu.5 chize.**

Location: at the level of elbow crease, on the lateral border of biceps tendon.

Indications: Pain and swelling of elbow, arthritis of elbow, skin diseases, asthma, haemoptysis.

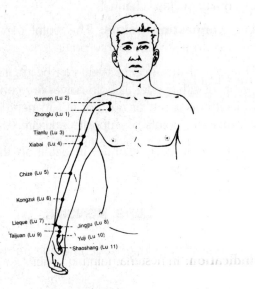

Lung Meridian

Needing 0.5 cun perpendicularly. Bleeding at this point and injecting the same drawn blood at GB30 helps effectively in psoriasis, eczema when pruritus is marked.

3. Lu.6 Kongzui

Location: 5 cun distal to Lu5 on the path of channel. It is located on the medial border of Radius. It is indicated in acute asthma, tonsilitis, acute rhinitis, bleeding haemorrhoids, aphonia etc. It is an important XI-cleft point and needling is done perpendicularly with a strong manual stimulation.

Lu.7 lieque: It is located 1.5 cun proximal; from the wrist joint crease on the outer, radial or lateral border of forearm.

Indications: In occipital headache, cervical spondylosis, lung disorders, skin diseases etc. It is a distal point for back of neck, head and back of lungs. Needle is directed proximally in proximal disorders, inserted distally in wrist joint diseases.

4. Lu.9 taiyuan:

Location: At the outer end of wrist crease on the lateral side of radial artery.

Indications: a. In wrist joint diseases b. Arteriosclerosis c. Vascular disorders d. Asthma e. Allergic and skin disorders.

Needling is done 0.3 cun perpendicularly avoiding radial artery. It is a Yuan source point and also an influential point for blood vessels.

5. Lu.11 Shao shang:

Location: It is located 0.1 cun proximal to the outer corner of the nail of thumb.

Indication: In hysteria, fainting epilepsy, convulsions, and acute emergencies including tonsillitis and epistaxis. Needle is inserted 0.1 cun perpendicular to cause bleeding or strong stimulation.

LARGE INTESTINE MERIDIAN L.I.

This meridian is connected to large intestine, lung, skin, nose and body hairs.

LI. 4 Hegu

Location: It is stimulated in the web between the forefinger and thumb on the dorsal aspect of hand at the top of 1st dorsal interosseous muscle in the adducted thumb.

Indications: a. Disorders of thumb, forefinger and wrist joint.

b. Distal point for front of head, face, special sense organs and front of neck.

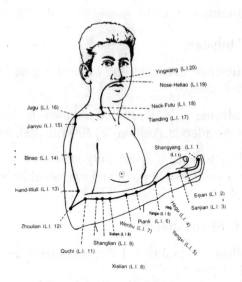

Large Intestine Meridian

c.   Disorders of lung.

d.   Yuan source point of large intestine.

e.   Upper extremity paralysis.

f.   One of the best analgesic points.

g.   Hyperhidrosis (Excessive perspiration)

Puncturing is done 0.5 to 1.0 cun perpendicularly.

LI. 10 Shousani I:

Location: On the lateral aspect of forearm 2.0 cun below LI. 11.

Indications: Tennis elbow, acupressure point for headache tumors etc.

Needle is inserted 1.0 to 1.5 cun perpendicularly.

LI. 11: Quchi.

Location: At the outer end of elbow crease in semiflexed elbow.

a. Tennis elbow.

b. Upper extremity paralysis.

c. Diabetes mellitus.

d. Hypertension.

p. Irregular menstruation.

f. Homoeostatic point and immune enhancing point.

LI. 16 Jianyu:

Location: At the anterior depression laternal to the tip of acromion process.

Indications: a. Capsulitis of shoulder

b. Neck spasm.

c. Paralysis upper extremity.

Needle is inserted 0.5 to 1.5 cun perpendicularly.

LI 18 neck futu.

Location: 3 cun lateral to adam's apple.

Indications: Vocal cord nodule, Goitre. sore throat asthma etc.

Puncturing is done 0.3 cun deep with moxa also.

LI. 19 nose (Helino)

Location: 0.5 cun lateral to point Du26 after the channel has crossed the midline.

Indications: Epistaxis, facial palsy, trigeminal neuralgia, coryza.

Needling is done 0.3 to 0.5 cun obliquely directed medially.

LI 20 (Ying xiang):

Location: In the horizontal line drawn from the outermost point of alae nasi on the nasolabial groove.

Indications: Epistaxis, nasal obstruction, Facial palsy and trigeminal neuralgia etc.

Puncture is 0.3 to 0.5 cun obliquely and directed medially.

L.I. Channel is the only channel which ends on the opposite side. LI19 and L.I.20 are on the opposite sides.

STOMACH MERIDIAN (ST.)

Stomach meridian is connected to stomach, spleen mouth and flesh of limbs. It is used mainly for local disorders.

St$_2$ SIBAI:

Location: 0.7 cun below midpoint of inferior orbital margin.

Indications: Facial palsy, eye diseases.

Needle is directed horizontally upwards

St$_3$. Julio.

Location: On the mid pupillary line below st2. At the level of alae nasi.

Indications: a. Facial palsy b. Trigeminal neuralgia.

c. Speech disorders d. toothhaches.

Needle is directed towards nose horizontally.

St$_4$ Dicang:

Location: 0.4 cun lateral to corner of mouth.

Indications: Facial palsy, excessive salivation, disorders of upper teeth.

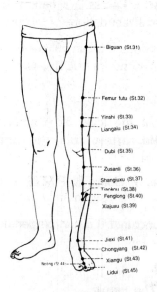

Biguan (St.31)

Femur futu (St.32)

Yinshi (St.33)
Liangqiu (St.34)

Dubi (St.35)

Zusanli (St.36)
Shangjuxu (St.37)
Tiaokou (St.38)
Fenglong (St.40)
Xiajuxu (St.39)

Jiexi (St.41)
Chongyang (St.42)
Xiangu (St.43)
Neiting (St.44)
Lidui (St.45)

Stomach Meridian

Needling is done horizontally upwards towards St. 6 for bell's palsy, while directed towards mouth for speech and salivation.

St₆ Jiache

Location: One finger breadth antero superior to the lower angle of mandible.

Indication: a. Trigeminal neuralgia b. Trismus c. Spasm neck. d. Bell's palsy. e. Parotitis.

Needle is directed horizontally towards St₆.

St₈ touwei.

Location: 5 cun lateral to midpoint of anterior hair line i.e. 3 cun above outer corner of eyebrow.

Indications: a. Excess lacrimation b. migraine c. frontal headache d. mental retardation e. epilepsy.

Puncturing is done 0.5 cun obliquely directed posteriorly for headache and anteriorly for eye diseases

St₉. Renying.

Location: At the level of Adam's apple, posterior to common carotid artery on the anterior border of sternocliedomastoid.

Indications: a. Goitre b. P.M.G. c. Flushing of face d. Asthma etc.

Needle is punctured 0.3 cun perpendicularly. Avoiding the site of artery.

St ₁₇: Ruzhong.

Location: The nipple.

Indications: It is prohibited: only moxa is allowed.

St 25 tianshu:

Location: 2 cun lateral to umbilicus.

Indications: a. Pain umbilical region around b. Paralytic ileus c. Obesity d. Flatulent Dyspepsia

It is a mu front alarm point of large intestines.

St 29. Guilai:

Location: 4 cun below St 25.

Indications: a. Impotence b. Azoospermia c. Uterine prolapse, d. menstrual irregularities e. Hernia etc.

Needle is directed horizontally downwards.

St 32 Femur.

Location: 6 cun above the outer bed of upper border of patella.

Indications: a. Paralysis of lower limb. (Hemiplegia) b. Muscular dystrophy. c. Pain Iliac region (non specific enteritis):

Needle is inserted 2 cun perpendicular. It is very effective for injection therapy where in hemiplegia it is of use in postpolio paralysis.

St34. Liangqiu:

Location: 2 cun above the outer end of upper border of patelia.

Indications: It is XI cleft point of stomach channel. Helpful in acute colicky abdomen needle is inserted 1 cun perpendicular with a strong manual stimulation. Fire needing technique is used for fluid retention or crystic knee joint.

St35. Dubi:

Location: On outer depression of knee with knee partially flexed.

Indication: Osteoarthritis of knees.

Needle is directed obliquely towards the centre of knee joint.

St36 (zusanli)

Location: 1. Finger breadth lateral to lower end of tibial tuberosity, 3 cun below St 35.

Indications: a. Osteoarthritis knees b. Diabetes c. Hypertension d. As a homoeostatic point.' e. Neuropathy. Facial palsy g. Bronchial asthma.

Needle is inserted 1 cun perpendicular, directed upwards for facial paralysis.

St 37 (Shang chushu)

Location: 3 cun distal to St 36,, 1 finger breadth lateral to shin of tibia.

Indications: a. Diarrhoea b. Acute appendicitis, c. Hemiplegia needle is inserted 1 cun perpendicular.

Ex 33 (Lanwei)

Location: 2 cun distal to St 36.

Indications: It is used as an alarm point in the diagnosis, treatment and prognosis of acute appendicitis.

Needled: 1.0 cun perpendicular.

This point was identified later so it is known as extra point although it lies on the pathway of St. meridian.

St 38 Thokou:

Location: 5.0 cun below St 36, 1 finger breadth lateral to the anterior border of tibia.

Indications: a. Frozen shoulder b. capsulitis of shoulder c. Spasm of Gastrocnemius muscle.

Needling is done vertically 1 cun. It is a magic point for frozen shoulder.

St$_{40}$ fenflong:

Location: 1. Finger breadth lateral to St 38.

Indications: a. Grandmal epilepsy b. Hemiplegia c. Asthma d. Bronchietasis e. Depressive neurosis.

Needle is inserted 1 cun vertical.

St $_{41}$ Jiexi:

Location: Midway between the malleoli on the anterior angle crease, between the tendons of extensor digitorum longus and hallucis longus

Indications: a. Vertigo b. Ankle joint disorders c. Oedema facial d. Headache, e. Cervical spondylosis.

St.44 neiting

Location: 0.5 cun above the web margin between 2nd and 3rd toes.

Indications: a. Epistaxis b. Tonsillitis, c. Fever d. Insomnia e. Analgesic point of facial palsy.

SPLEEN MERIDIAN

It is connected to spleen, stomach, pancreas, mouth and flesh of limbs

Sp.3: Yinbai:

Location: 0.1 cun posterior to medial corner of base of nail of great toe.

Indications: a. Leucorrhoea. b. Abdominal distension c. Menorrhagia d. Convulsions.

Needling is done 0.1 cun obliquely.

Sp.6 San Yin Jiao:

Location: 3 cun above the tip of medial malleolus, posterior to the border of tibia.

Indications: a. Angioneurotic oedema. b. Homoeostatic, tonification and immune enhancing point. c. Diabetes mellitus. d. Impotence. e. Used as a distal point for oligo spermia, Azoospermia etc. f. Insomnia. Sp 9. (Yinlingqvan)

Location: At the level of lower border of tibial tuberosity in the depression below the lower border of medial condyle.

Indications: a. Oedema and ascites b. Irregular menstruation. c. O.A. Knees.

Puncture 1.5 cun perpendicular.

Sp.10 Zue hai

Location: 2 cun above the medial end of upper border of patella.

Indications: a. Ulticaria b. D.U.B. (Dysfunctional uterine bleeding) c. O.A. knees.

Needle is inserted 1.5 cun perpendicularly.

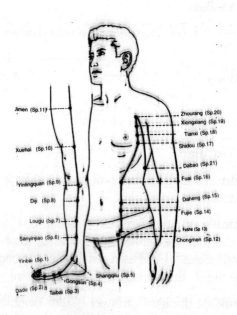

Jimen (Sp.11)

Zhourang (Sp.20)
Xiongxiang (Sp.19)
Tianxi (Sp.18)

Xuehai (Sp.10)

Shidou (Sp.17)

Dabao (Sp.21)

Yinlingquan (Sp.9)

Fuai (Sp.16)

Diji (Sp.8)

Daheng (Sp.15)

Fujie (Sp.14)

Lougu (Sp.7)

Fushe (Sp.13)

Sanyinjiao (Sp.6)

Chongmen (Sp.12)

Yinbai (Sp.1)

Shangqiu (Sp.5)

Gongsun (Sp.4)

Dadu (Sp.2)

Taibai (Sp.3)

Spleen Meridian-I

Sp.15 Daheng.

Location: 4 cun lateral to umbilicus

Indications: a. Constipation b. Paralytic ileus. c. Ascariasis.

It regulates the activites of stomach and intestines.

Needling 1.0 cun perpendicular.

Sp.16 Fuai:

Location: 3 cun above daheng.

Indications: a. Abdominal distension and pain. b. Ascariasis:

Needling is done 1.0 cun perpendicular.

HEART MERIDIAN

Heart meridian is connected to heart, small intestine, tongue, brain and blood vessels:

H.3 Shaohai

Location: Medial end of elbow crease when the elbow is fully flexed.

Indications: a. Numbness of upper limb. b. Lymphadenitis (Axilla) c. Tennis elbow.

H.5 Tongli

Location: 1.0 cun proximal to H_7 on the radial side of tendon of flexor carpii ulnaris.

Indication: a. Aphasia b. Hoarseness voue c. S t a m - mering

Needling is done 0.5 cun perpendicular.

H.6 Yinxi.

Location: 0.5 cun proximal to H_7.

Indications: a. Hyperhidrosis b. Non specific intercostal neuralgia

Punctured 0.5 cun perpendicular.

It is an important Xi-cleft point.

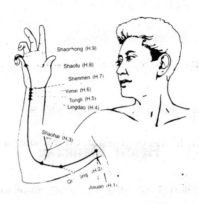

The Three levels of energy

Heart Meridian

H.7 shenmen:

Location: On the radial side of tendon of flexor carpi ulnaris at wrist crease.

Indications: a. Palpitation. b. Hysteria c. Insomnia d. Epilepsy. e. Cerebral palsy.

Needing is 0.5 cun perpendicular.

H.8 Shao chong:

Location: 0.1 cun proximal to the radial corner of the nail of little finger.

Indications: a. Apoplexy b. Palpitation.

0.5 cun perpendicularly. It is a marked Jingwell point.

SMALL INTESTINE

This meridian is connected to small intestine, heart, brain, blood vessels and tongue.

Points are used mainly for local and neck disorders.

S.I 3. Houx I

Location: At the medial end of main transverse crease of palm on clenching the wrist.

Indications: a. Cervical spasm. b. Torticollis c. L.B.A. d. Intercostal neuralgia.

Needing is 0.5 cun perpendicular with strong manual stimulation.

S.I 6 Yang lad:

Location: In the depression on the lateral aspect of styloid process of ulna.

Indications: a Wrist pain. b. Cervical spondylosis c. Intercostal neuralgia. d. Hemiplegia.

Needle is inserted 1.0 cun obliquely towards P6.

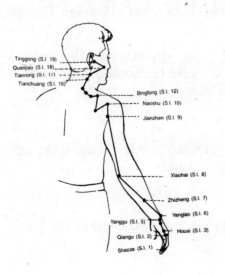

Small Intestine Meridian

S.I 9 Jhan Zhen.

Location: 1.0 cun superior to the highest point of posterior axillary fold.

Indications: a. Frozen shoulder. b. Hemiplegia c. Toothache. d. High fevers.

Needle is inserted 1.5 cun perpendicular.

S.I 18 Quanliao

Location: In the depression below the prominence of Zygomatic bone on a vertical line drawn from the outer canthus of eye.

Indications: a. Twitching of eyelids. b. Trigeminal neuralgia. c. Facial paralysis. d. Used as an analgesic point in tooth extraction, and minor surgical interventions.

Needle is inserted 0.3 to 0.5 cun perpendicular.

S.I 14 Tinggong:

Location: In the depression felt between tragus and mandibular joint in half open mouth

Indications: a. Deafness b. Menerier's Disease c. Chronic otitis media

Needle is inserted 0.5 cun perpendicular. This point is punctured along with S.I 21, GB2 Horizontally downwards. It is called "Puncture through technique"

Urinary bladder (U.B)

This meridian is closely related to U.B. kidney, scalp, hair bone, cartilage, ear and sex organs.

U.B2 Zanzhu:

Location: At the depression of medial end of eye brow, directly above the inner canthus.

Indications: a. Blepharitis b. Frontal sinusitis.

U.B 11 Dashu: This is an influential point for bones and cartilage.

Location: 1.5 cun laternal to the lower border of spinous process of T_1.

Indications: a. Osteo and rheumatoid arthritis, cervical spondylosis.

U.B13 Feishu: It is the back shu point of lung.

Location: 1.5 cun lateral to the lower border of spinous process of T_3.

Indications a. Rhinitis b. Bronchitis.

Intercostal Neuralgia.

Needling is done 0.3 - 0.5 cun perpendicularly or obliquely downwards.

U.B 15 Xinshu: Back shu point of heart.

Location: 1.5 cun lateral to the lower border of spinous process of T5.

Indications: a. Hysteria b. Epilepsy, c. Insomnia d. Behavioural disorders.

Needle is inserted 0.3 to 0.5 cun perpendicularly or obliquely.

U.B 17 Geshy: Influential point for blood, and back shu point for diaphragm.

Location: 1.5 cun lateral to the lower border of spinous process of T_7.

Indications: a. Hiccough b. Urticaria. c. A n o r e x i a nervosa d. Chronic haemorrhagic tendencies.

0.3 to 0.5 cun perpendicular or obliquely downwards.

U.B 23 Shenshu   Back shu point of kidney.

Location: 1.5 cun lateral to the lower border of spinous process of L2.

Indications: a. Genito urinary disorders. b. Alopecia c. Impotency d. Chronic lumbago.

Needle is inserted 1.0 cun perpendicular or obliquely towards vertebral column.

U.B 25 Dachangshu:

Back shu point of large intestine.

Location: 1.5 cun lateral to the lower border of spinous process of L_4 vertebrae.

Indications: a. Sciatica b. Diarrhoea c. Haemorrhoids.

Punituring: 1.0 - 1.5 cun. Perpendicular.

U.B 32 Ciliao:

Location: 2nd sacral foramina.

Indications: a. Irregular menses. b. Urgency of micturition.

Needle is inserted 0.5 cun perpendicular.

U.B 36 (Chengfu)

Location: In the middle of gluteal fold.

Indications: a. Sciatica b. Hemiplegia, c. Occipital headache.

Needle is inserted 2.3 cun perpendicular.

U.B 40 Wei zhong:

Location: At the midpoint of popliteal transverse crease.

Indications: a. Sciatica b. Lumbago. c. Sunstroke d. Contracted calf muscles write neuralgia.

Needle is inserted 0.5 to 1.0 cun perpendicular or prick to bleed in skin diseases.

U.B 54 Zhibian.

Location: At the level of 4th sacral folamen, 3 cun lateral to midline

Indications: a. A vascular necrosis of hip joints (A.V.N.) b. Sciatica c. Rectal prolapse.

Needle is inserted 1.5 to 2.0 cun perpendicular.

U.B 56 chengjin

Location: 5 cun below U.B 40.

Indications: Calf muscle spasm.

Puncturing: 1.5 cun perpendicular.

U.B 57 Yinmen.

Location: 6.0 cun distal to U.B 36 on a line joining U.B 36 and U.B 40.

Location: At the level where two bellies of Gastrocnemius muscles unite to form tendo achillies, 8 cun below U.B 40 or halfway between U.B 40 and ankle joint.

Indications: a. Sciatica b. Plantar fascitis c. Haemorrhoids d. Rectal prolapse e. Anal fissure.

Needle is inserted 1.0 to 1.5 cun perpendicularly.

U.B 60 Kunluid

Location: Lies midway between the prominence of lateral malleous and lateral border of tendo achillies

Indications: a. Sciatica b. Cervical spasm c. Epistaxis d. Lumbago chronic

Needling is done 0.5 - 0.8 cun perpendicular.

U.B 62 Shenmai.

Locations: 0.5 cun inferior to the tip of lateral malleolus.

Indications: a. Convulsions b. Epilepsy c. Foot drop d. Drug deaddiction.

It is one of the most important sedative and tranquilizing point of lower limb.

Needle is inserted 0.3 to 0.5 cun.

U.B 67 Zhiyin.

Location: 0.1 cun proximal to the lateral end of base of nail of little toe.

Indications: a. Difficult labour. b. Epistaxis c. Blurring of vision.

Needle is inserted 0.1 cun perpendicularly heating the upper half of needle with moxa is highly effective.

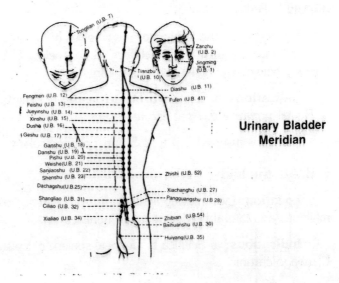

Urinary Bladder Meridian

KIDNEY MERIDIAN

It is connected to kidney, urinary bladder, bone , cartilages, ear, sex organs and scalp hairs.

K.1 Yongquan

Location: It lies on a point between 2nd and 3rd toes. In the depression between the anterior one third and posterior two third of plantar flexed sole.

Indications: a. Shock, hysteria b. Hyperemesis gravidarum c. Used as a jingwell point in coma, Faints and hysteria. d. Hyperhidrosis e. Hypertension

Needle is intserted 0.5 cun perpendicular and prick to bleed in emergency

K.3 taixi.

Location: Midway between the tip of medial malleolus and medial border of tendo achilles.

Indications: a. U.T.I. b. L.B.A. c. Impotence, d. Acute asthmatic attack. e. Deafness f. Noctural enuresis.

Needle is inserted 1.0 cun perpendicular

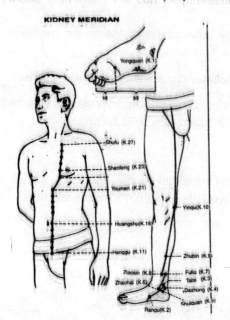

KIDNEY MERIDIAN

Yongquan (K.1)

Kidney Meridian

Shufu (K.27)

Shenfeng (K.23)

Youmen (K.21)

Yingu(K.10)

Huangshu(K.16)

Henggu (K.11)

Zhubin (K.9)

Zhaoxin (K.8)

Fuliu (K.7)

Zhaohai (K.6)

Taixi (K.3)

Dazhong (K.4)

Shuiquan (K.5)

Rangu(K.2)

K.7 Fuliu

Location: 2 cun proximal to K3 on the medial border of tendo achilles.

Indications: a. Hair fall   b. Hyperhidrosis. c. Deafness d. Pedal oedema and ascites.

K.10 Yingu:

Location: At the popliteal crease on the medial border of semitendinosus

Indications: a. Alopecia areata. b. Dysuria c. D.U.B. d. Impotence.

Needle is inserted 1.0 cun perpendicular.

PERICARDIUM MERIDIAN

It is known as Xin Pao luo jing called as circulation. Sex and heart constrictor. It starts 1 cun lateral to the nipple, runs, along the front of upper limb between the lung channel and heart channel and ends at the tip of middle finger.

P.3 Quze

Location: In the ante cubital crease on the medial border of biceps tendon.

Indications: Palpitation, anxiety, angina pectoris.

Needle: Is inserted 1.0 cun perpendicular. In case of high fever, bleeding with 3 edged needle is helpful.

P.4 Ximen

Location: 5 cun proximal to the midpoint of the wrist crease, between the tendons of palmaris longus and flexor carpii Radialis muscle.

Indications: a. Tachycardia of psycogenic origin b. Sinus arrythmia. c. Hysteria. d. Acute depressive neurosis.

It is a Xi-Cleft point.

Needle is inserted 1.0 cun perpendicularly.

P.6 Neigun: It is one of the six significant luo connecting and distal points.

Location: 2.0 cun proximal to the midpoint of wrist crease, between the tendons of palmaris longus and flexor carpi radialis.

Indications: a. Pericarditis b. Brain disorders.

eg: Epilepsy, hysteria, Insomnia etc. c. Distal point for chest and abdominal   disorders eg. Hyper-emesis, Peptic ulcer syndrome etc. d. Numbness of forearm and hands. e. For Acupuncture anaesthesia and cardiac surgery f. Thyroidectomy.

Needle is inserted 1.0 cun perpendicular.

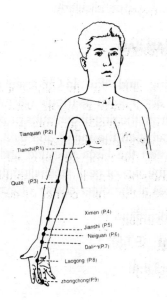

Pericardium Meridian

P.7 Daling: It is a yuan source point.

Location: At the midpoint of wrist crease between the tendons of palmaris longus and flexur carpi radialis.

Indications: a. Diseases of wrist joint. b. Median nerve compression. c. Carpal tunnel syndrome.

Needle is inserted 0.5 cun perpendicularly.

In diseases of wrist joint this point is usually combined with H.7 and Lu.9.

P.8. Laogong:

Location: In the palmar surface between the tips of middle and ring fingers as they touch the centre of palm on clenching the fist.

Indications: 1. Disorders of palm. 2. Rheumatoid Arthritis. 3. Duptyren's, Contracture. 4. Hyper Hidrosis.

Needle is inserted 0.5 cun perpendicularly.

SANJIAO

It is the protector of "Zang" and "Fu". In Chinese it means **three body cavities.** It is also known as tripple warmer and three burning space. It starts from the ring finger, runs proximally on the back of upper limb between the radius and ulna, more or less parallel to and between the large intestine and small intestine channels. It runs to the side of neck, encircling the root of external ear and terminates at the outer corner of eyebrow.

Related channel: Pericardium.

Luo connecting point: (S.I.5)

Yuan source point: (S.J.4)

S. J3 Zhongzhu

Location on the dorsum of hand in the depression between the heads of 4th and 5th metacarpal bones. It is located by fist clenching.

Indications: 1. Ear disorders. 2. Hemiplegia.

Needle is inserted perpendicular.

S.J 5 Waigun.

Location: 2 cun proximal to the midpoint of dorsal transverse crease of wrist between radius and ulna.

Indications: a. Hemiplegia b. Hypertension. c. Otitis media d. Wryneck.

Needle is inserted 1.0 cun perpendicular.

S.J 6 Zhigou

Location: 1.0 cum proximal to waigun.

Indications: a. Constipation.

Needle is inserted 1.0 cun perpendicular.

S.J8 Sanyangluo:

Location: 1.0 cun proximal to zhigou.

Indications: a. Intercostal neuralgia. b. Acupuncture anaesthesia for throat surgery.

Needle is inserted 1.0 cun perpendicular

S.J. 14 (Jianliao)

Location: In abducted arm, in the posterior depression of origin of deltoid muscles, from the lateral border of acromion process. with the arm by the side between the acromion and greater tuberosity of humerus.

Indications: a. Hemiplegia b. Paralysis. c. Myalgia.

Needling is done 1.0 cun perpendicular towards H.7.

S.J. 17 (Y1 Feng)

Location: In the highest point of depression behind the ear lobe between the angle and the mastoid process.

Indications: a. Otitis media. b. Facial palsy.

Needle is inserted 1.0 cun perpendicular.

S.J 20 (Jiasun)

Location: On the scalp at ear apex, when ear is folded forwards.

Indications: a. Endocrinal disorders specially of pituitary origin. eg. Drawfism. Needle is inserted 0.5 cun obliquely downwards.

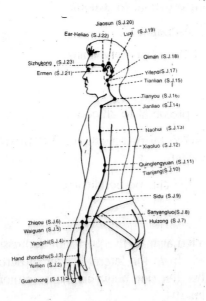

Sanjiao Meridian

S.J 21 (Ermen)

Location: In the depression in front of supra tragic notch. It is located when the mouth is slightly open.

Indications: Ear disorders.

Needling is done 0.5 cun perpendicular.

SJ. 23 (Sizhukong)

Location: In the depression at the lateral end of eyebrow.

Indications: a. Eye disorders. b. Temporal and frontal headache.

Needle is inserted horizontally and posteriorly in the direction of GB_8.

GALL BLADDER MERIDIAN

It is appended to liver and they mutually assist one another to perform their functions. It runs from head to foot on the lateral aspect of body. It starts from the outer corner of eye and runs to the front of ear. It then Zig Zags over the side of head, from the posterolateral aspect of trunk and the lower limb to the end of foot near the lateral corner of the base of 4th toe nail.

This meridian is related to gall bladder, liver, muscles, tendon and eyes.

G.B 2 (Tinghui)

Location: In the depression immediately in front of inter tragic north when mouth is open.

Indications: a. Deafness b. Otitis media c. Chronic ear infections. d. Arthritis affecting mandible. e. Facial palsy f. Parotitis.

Needle is inserted 1.0 cun perpendicular

G.B 8 (Shyaigu)

Location: Directly above the apex of ear, 1.5 cun above the hair line.

Indications: a. Cerebral palsy b. Migraine c. Infantile convulsions.

Needling is 1.0 cun horizontally anteriorly for headache, upwards for brain disorders, downwards for ear disorders.

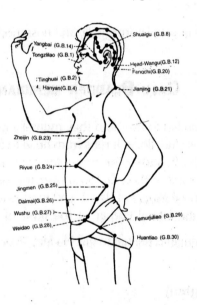

Gall Bladder Meridian

G.B 14 Yang bai:

Location: 1.0 cun above the midpoint of eyebrow.

Indications: a. Facial palsy b. Frontal sinusitis c. Nyctalopia d. Optic atrophy, c. Twitching of eyelids.

Needling is 0.5 cun horizontally and inferiorly towards Ex3.

G.B 20. (Fengchi)

Location: In the depression medial to mastoid process between the origin of trapezius and sternomastoid muscles.

Indications: a. Occipital headache b. coryza c. Cervical spondylosis d. Optic atrophy e. Progressive myopia.

Needle is inserted 1.0 cun directed towards inner canthus of the opposite eye:

G.B 21 (Jian jing)

Location: It is midway between Du_{14} and LI_{15} ie. midway between 7th cervical vertebra and acromion process.

Indications: a. It is an alarm point for gall bladder. b. Capsulitis shoulder   c. Ankylosing spondylitis

d. D.U.B. e. Endocrine and metabolic disorders.

Needle is inserted 1.0 cun perpendicular.

G.B 30 (Huantiao)

Location: Draw a straight line between the highest point of greater trochanter and the sacral hiatus. It is situated at the junction of our third with junction of outer third with the middle two third on the line.

Indications: a. Sciatica b. Prolapsed lumbar disc. c. Hemiplegia d. LBA. Needle is inserted perpendicularly. It is highly beneficial in acute sciatica

G.B 31 (Feng shi)

Location: On the lateral aspect of thigh 7 cun proximal to the popliteal crease, between vastus lateralis and femoral muscles. This can be located in standing position with the middle finger touching the lateral aspect of thigh.

Indications: a. Hemiplegia b. Post polio paralysis c. Neuropathy

Needle is inserted 1.5 cun perpendicular.

G.B 34 (Yangling quan)

Location: In the depression anterior and inferior to the head of fibula

Indications: a. Hemiplegia b. Paraplegia c. Chole cystitis. d. Epilepsy. e. neck strain.

It is the influential point for muscles and tendons. Needle is inserted 1.5 cun perpendicular towards sp 9. Or obliquely downwards, forwards and medially.

G.B 37 (Guang mind)

Locations: 5 cun above the tip of lateral malleolus on the anterior border of fibula.

Indications. a. Conjunctivitis. b. Headache.

Needle is inserted 1.0 cun perpendicular. It is a luo connecting point.

G.B. 39 Xuan zhong.

Location: 3 cun above the tip of lateral malleolus on the posterior border of firula

Indications: a. Hemiplegia b. Cervical spondylosos. c. Hypertension d. Intercostal neuralgia.

Needle is inserted 1.0 cun perpendicular. It is the influential point of bone marrow.

G.B 41 Foot linqi.

Location: In the depression immediately distal to the junction of base of 4th and 5th metatarsals.

Indications: a. Breast disorders b. Plantar fascitis c. Otitis media, It is a supplementary point for frozen shoulder.

Needle is inserted 0.5 cun perpendicular.

G.B 43 Zia xi

Location: 0.5 cun proximal to the web margin between 4th and 5th toes

Indications: a. Blurring of vision. b. Deafness c. Secondary Amenorrhoea. Needle is inserted 0.5 cun obliquely.

LIVER MERIDIAN

This channel is related to liver, gall bladder, muscles, tendon and eyes.

Liv. 3 (Tai chong)

Location: 2.0 cun proximal to the web margin of 1st and 2nd toes.

Indications: a. Hypertension b. Chronic hepatitis c. Insomnia d. Diabetes mellitus e. Schizophrenia.

Needle is inserted 1.0 cun obliquely in a proximal direction.

It is a yuan source point as well as a good homoeostatic point.

Liv. 6 Zhongdu.

Location: 7 cun superior to the tip of medial malleolus on the medial border of tibia.

Indications: a. Pelvic inflammatory disease. b. chronic vaginitis c. Irregular menses. d. Cholecystitis and cholelithiasis

It is an alarm point of liver.

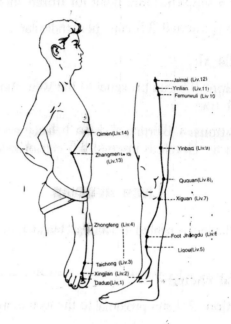

Jaimai (Liv.12)
Yinlian (Liv.11)
Femurwuli (Liv 10
Qimen(Liv.14)
Zhangmen (a.13)
(Liv.13)
Yinbao (Liv.9)
Ququan(Liv 8),
Xiguan (Liv.7)
Zhongfeng (Liv.4)
Foot Jhangdu (Liv 6
Ligou(Liv.5)
Taichong (Liv.3)
Xingjian (Liv.2)
Dadun(Liv.1)

Liver Meridian

Liv. 8 Ququan

Location: In the transverse crease of joint at the medial border of semimembranous tendon.

Indications: a. O.A. Knees b. Uterine prolapse c. Impotence. d. U.T.I.

Needle is inserted 1.0 cun.

Liv. 13 Zhangmen

Location: On the lateral side of abdomen below the free end of floating rib.

Indications: a. Non specific gastritis. b. Hepatitis

It is the influential point for solid organs.

Needle is inserted 0.5 cun deep

DU Meridian or Governing vessel

This is related to brain, bone marrow, kidney, uterus, nose, eyes, mouth and lips.

DU3 Yaoyang guag.

Location: On the back midline between the dorsal spine of L4 & L5; at the upper border of Iliac crest.

Indications: a. L.B.A. b. Genito urinary disorder c. Impotence d. Leucorrhoea. Needle is inserted 1.o cun perpendicular.

DU4 (Mingmen)

Location: On the back midline between the dorsal spines of T_{11} and T_{12}.

Indications: a. Diarrhoea b. Epilepsy c. Haemorrhoids. This point causes relaxation in spastic states.

Needle is inserted 0.5 cun obliquely upwards.

DU8 Zhiyang

Location: Below the spinous process of T7

Indications: a. Cholecystitis b. Jaundice c. L.B.A.

Needle is inserted 1.0 cun deep.

DU 11 (Shendao)

Location: On the back midline between the dorsal spines of T_5 & T_6.

Indications: a. Loss of memory b. Depressive neurosis c. Anxiety neurosis needle is directed obliquely upwards 0.5 cun.

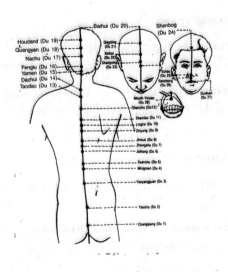

DU Meridian

DU14 Dazhui.

Location: On the back midline between the dorsal spines of C_7 & T_1 vertebrae.

Indications: a. Epilepsy b. Migraine c. Cervical spondylosis d. Torticollis e. It is the most important immune enhancing point thereby improving and tonifying the homoeostasis all body. f. Lung disorders: Cough, bronchial asthma etc. g. Haemorrhoids.

Needle is inserted 1.0 cun perpendicular.

DU 15 (Yamen)

Location: At the midpoint of nape of neck 0.5 cun within the posterior hair line.

Indications: a. Deaf mutism b. Cervical spondylosis c. C.V.A. d. Schizophrenia.

Needling is 1.0 cun obliquely towards throat.

DU 16 Fengfu

Location: 0.5 cun above Du 15.

Indications: Similar to Du 15.

Needle is inserted 1.0 cun obliquely towards adam apple. Deep insertion is risky.

DU 18 Qiangjian

Location: Midway between Du 16 $ Du 29,

Indications: a. Occipital hedache b. Neck Rigidity.

Needle is inserted 0.5 cun horizontally.

DU 20 Baihui

Location: a. Draw a straight line from the tip of ear lobe to the apex of auricle and extend this line upwards on the scalp till it intersects the midline. The point lies at this intersection. b. On the vertex of skull, 5 cun behind anterior hair line and 7.0 cun above the posterior hair line in the midline. c. On the midline 8 cun behind the glabella. d. On the midline 7.0 cun above the posterior hair line in the midline. c. On the midline 8 cun behind the glabella. d. On the midline 7.0 cun above the posterior hair line.

Indications: 1. One of the best sedative and tranquilizing point. 2. Cerebral palsy & mental retardation. 3. Amnesia. 4. Impotence 5. Bronchial asthma. 6. Alopecia areata. 7. Used as a distal point for haemorrhoids and rectal prolapse.

Needle is directed 0.3 to 0.5 cun obliquely or horizontally with the needle directed posteriorly. No electro stimulation.

D.U 26 (Renzhong)

Location: At the junction of upper third and lower two thirds of philtrum of the upper lip midline.

Indications: a. Jingwell point for acute emergencies like epileptic fit, fainting, heat stroke b. Distal point for L.B.A. c. Facial palsy d. Rhinitis e. Epistaxis.

Needle is inserted 0.3 to 0.5 cun obliquely backwards and upwards. In emergency bleeding at this point helps in revival.

Important: 1. It is used as a reanimation point in the emergency treatment. 2. It is the meeting point of 3. Yang channels.

3. Dr. Lohia has used it successfully in acute cardiac pain by applying firm nail pressure at this point.

REN MERIDIAN OR CONCEPTIONAL VESSEL

Uterus, lips and eyes are related organs.

Ren.2 Qugu:

Location: At the middle of upper border of symphysis pubis ie. 5 cun below the umbilicus

Indications: a. Incontinence b. Seminal emissions. c. Chronic pelvic inflammatory disease. d. Irregular menstruation.

Needle is directed horizontally downwards.

Ren. zhongji:

Location: In the front midline 4 cun below the umbilicus.

Indications: a. Genitourinary disorders b. Nocturnal enuresis c. P.I.D. d. Impotence.

Needle is directed 1.5 cun perpendicular or obliquely. It is the alarm point of urinary bladder.

Ren.4 Guanyan:

Location: In the front midline, 3 cun below the umbilicus.

Indications: a. Incontinence b. Nocturnal enuresis c. Hyperacidity.

Needle is inserted 1.0 cun perpendicular.

It is the alarm point of small intestine.

Ren.5 shimen:

Location: In the front midline 2 cun below the umbilicus.

Indications: a. Oedema and ascites b. Dysuria c. vague abdominal pains.

Needle is inserted 1.5 cun perpendicular.

It is the alarm point of sanjiao and can be used in oedema and ascites with Ren_9, sp_9 and UB_{20}.

Ren.6 Qihas:

Location: In the front midline 1.5 cun below the umbilicus.

Indications: a. Neurasthenia b. Diarrhoea

It is a tonification point and used for chronic fatigue and hypotension.

c. Asthma d. Impotence.

Needle is inserted 1.5 cun perpendicular.

Ren.8 shenjue:

Location: Centre of umbilicus.

Indications: It is prohibited for acupuncture.

But used as an anatomical landmark to locate other points. Diarrhoea is treated by moxibustion at this point. Cupping is also beneficial.

Ren.9 Shuifen

Location: In the front midline 1.0 cun above the umbilicus.

Indications: a. P.U.S. b. Abdominal distension c. Non specific dyspepsia. It is an alarm point of stomach and influential point for hollow organs.

Needle is inserted 1.5 cun perpendicularly.

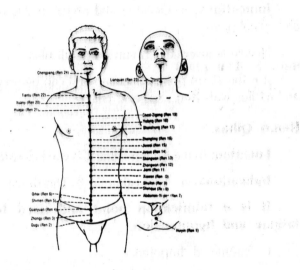

Ren Meridian

Ren.17 Shanzhong

Location: On the sternum midway between the two nipples.

Indications: a. Asthma b. Chest pain intervascular neuralgia c. Hiccough d. Dysphagia. e. Agalactia.

Needle is inserted 1.0 cun horizontally downwards. In breast disorders, the needle may be directed laterally, towards the diseased breast.

It is an alarm point of pericardium and influential point for lung tissue.

Ren.22 (Tiantu)

Location: In the centre of suprasternal dorsa, 0.5 cun above the sternal notch.

Indications: a. Bronchial asthma b. Hiccough c. Aphasia d. Dysphagia e. Goitre.

Needle is inserted 0.3 cun perpendicularly it is one of the dangerous points.

Ren.23 (Lianquan)

Location: On the midline of neck midway between adam's apple and lower border of mandible.

Indications: a. Aphasia b. Dyscrasia. c. Cerebral ataxia d. Dysphagia e. Chronic pharyngitis f. hyperhydrosis g. Tremors in parkinsonism.

Needle is inserted 1.0 to 1.5 cun obliquely towards the root of tongue towards Du 20.

Ren.24 Cheng Jiang.

Location: On the middle of mento labial groove, in the depression between the midpoint of chin and midpoint of lower lip.

Indications: a. Facial palsy b. Gingivitis c. Odontalgia d. Trigeminal neuralgia. e. As an anaesthetic point in tooth extraction.

It is the colliding point of Ren, Du and Yangming Meridians of both foot and hand and used as an excellent sedative and a tranquilizer point.

Needle is inserted 0.3 to 0.5 cun obliquely deep or horizontally 0.2 to 0.3 cun deep.

EXTRA POINTS (EX)

These points were numbered after the channels were already named.

Ex.1 (Yintang)

Location: On nasal ridge midway between the medial ends of two eye brows. It lies on Du channel.

Indications: a. Headache b. Dizziness c. Sinusitis d. Epileptic seizures e. Insomnia f. Allergic conjunctivitis.

Needle is inserted 0.5 cun horizontally downwards. Moxibustion is useful.

Ex.2 Taiyang:

Location: In the depression, about 1 cun posterior to the midpoint between the lateral ends of eyebrows and outer canthus of eye.

Indications: a migraine b. Trigeminal neuralgia c. Facial palsy d. Toothache.

Needle is directed 0.3 to 0.5 cun deep or prick to cause bleeding.

Ex.3 Yuyao:

Location: At the midpart of eyebrow.

Indications: a. Allergic blepharitis b. Ptosis c. Orbital spasm.

Needle is directed 0.3 to 0.5 cum laterally or inferiorly towards either side of eyebrow along the skin. Moxibustion is contra indicated

Ex.5 Juachengjiang:

Location: 1 cun lateral to Ren 24.

Indications: a Facial paralysis b. Chronic gingivitis c. Trigeminal neuralgia d. Toothache.

Puncturing is done 0.5 cun obliquely.

Ex.6 Sishen cong.

Location: Group of 4 points on the vertex one cun respectively, anterior, posterior and lateral to Du 20.

Indications: a. Cervical spondylosis. b. Insomnia c. Vertigo d. Mental retardation e. Epilepsy etc.

It **accelerates the action of Du 20.**

Ex.7 Yiming:

Location: 1. cun posterior to S. J 17.

Indications: Ear and eye disorders.

Needling is 0.5 cun perpendicularly

Ex.8 Anmian I:

Location: 0.5 cun posterior to S.J. 17

Indications: a. Cervical spondylitis b. Palpitation c. Anxiety neurosis d. Deaf mutism e. hysteria.

Ex.8 Anmian II:

Location: Midway between Ex. 7 and G B20

Indications: Similar to Ex. 8

Ex.10 Jin Jin:

Location: On the sublingual veins on either side of the root of tongue.

Indications: a. Aphthous stomatitis b. Pharyngitis. c. Gastroenteritis.

Needling is done with a three edged needle. It is contraindicated in haemophilia.

Ex. 17 Ding chuan.

Location: 0.5 cun lateral to Du 14.

Indications: a. Bronchial asthma b. Colicky abdominal pains.

Puncturing is done 0.5 cun obliquely directed medially.

Ex. 21 Huatuojiaji:

Location: Jia means besides and Ji means spinal column. The 17 points in this group are located 0.5 cun lateral to lower border of spinous process of vertebrae T1 to L5.

Indications: a. Jlaji points of upper back are used for diseases of heart, lungs and upper limbs. Jiaji points of lumbar region are used for disorders of lumbar region and lower limbs.

Jiaji points at the liver of back shu points can be used for ankilosing spondylitis and local disorders.

Ex. 28 Baxie: It is also known as Baguan de 8 weeks.

Location: 0.5 cun proximal to the web margin between the fingers.

Indications: a. Numbness at the tips of fingers b. Cervical spasm c. Viral fever.

Needle is directed 0.5 cun obliquely or prick to bleed.

Ex. 30 Yaoqi

Location: 2.0 cun above the coccyx.

Indications: a. Coccygeal pain b. Epilepsy.

Needle is inserted 1.0 cun obliquely directed upwards.

Ex. 31 Heding

Location: In the depression at the midpoint of upper border of patella when the knee is flexed.

Indications: a. Osteoarthrosis of knees b. Beriberi.

Needle is directed 0.5 cun perpendicular.

Ex. 32 Medial Xian

Location: Depression on the medial side of patellar ligament, when knee is fully flexed.

Indications: a. Osteoarthrosis knees b. Elephantiasis when limb pain is intolerable.

Needle is directed 0.5 to 1.0 cun deep towards the centre of knee joint.

Ex. 33. Lanwei:

Location: 2.0 cun distal to St 36 on the pathway of stomach meridian. Find out the maximum tender point.

Indications: a. Peptic ulcer syndrome b. Indigestion c. Appendicitis d. Early muscular dystrophy of Duchenn's type.

Needling is 1.0 cun perpendicular.

Ex. 35 Dannang

Location: 1.0 cun below G B 34

Indications: a. Cholecystitis

Needle is inserted 1.0 cun deep, perpendicular.

Ex. 36 Bafeng.

Location: 0.5 cun proximal to the web margin between the toes.

Indications: a. Pain at the dorsal fool. b. Headache c. Irregular menstruation.

Directed needle is 0.5 cun obliquely or prick to bleed.

MEDICAL ACUPUNCTURE

Till now we have discussed all possible, relevant details of acupuncture which are useful for us to arrive at a conclusion that acupuncture is also one of the auxillary techniques which is trying to establish it's roots gradually in the nomenclature of modes of treatment. Let us now discuss the practical applicability of acupuncture in context to arithritis in details. The therapeutic application of acupuncture is nothing but medical acupuncture.

In traditional Chinese medicine rheumatoid arthritis comes under Bi syndrome. It is a highly common and serious type of polyarthritis. Bi syndromes includes diseases like rheumatoid arthritis, rheumatic arthritis, neuralgia, Gout. Fibrositis etc. Bi sundrome is characterised by obstruction of Q1 $ Blood in meridians and collaterals due to invasion of pathogenic wind, cold and damp. Clinically, they are common in area where weather is cold, wet or windy. Long standing Bi Syndrome may turn into heat Bi, as the pathogenic factor in the meridians and collaterials are converted into heat.

These syndromes can be classified into:

a. **Wandering Bi:** Fleeting pains with polyarthritis, limitations of movements, fever of low grade type. Wandering pain is mainly due to invasion by pathogenic wind which is specialised by movement and changes.

b. **Painful Bi:** Severe pains relieved by heat and aggravated by cold without any local signs of inflammation. It is caused primarily by cold pathogenic factor which causes stagnation of blood with reflex vaso constriction.

c. **Fixed Bi:** Heaviness is the main feature caused by dampness. Numbness with heaviness of joints with aggravation on cloudy, rainy days.

d. **Heat Bi:** Heat converting pathogen is the prime factor. Initial features of acute inflammation with rapid pulse, fluctuating fever and complete immobility of joint is the prime feature.

e. **Vessel Bi:** Pain due to vascular blockage.

f. **Skin Bi:** Skin numb with coldness.

g. **Muscle Bi:** Sore and painful muscles.

h. **Bone Bi:** Pain only on movements or joints.

General principle of treatment: Aim of treatment is to eliminate the pathogenic factors like heat, wind, cold etc. thereby improving he circulation and allowing free flow of Qi.

GENERAL POINTS; FOR THE TREATMENT:

1. **Wandering pains:**
   a. Sp10, b. U.B 17; c. L.I.4; d. D U 14 e P.6
2. **Fixed Bi**
   a. St36　b. Sp6 C. L.I 4
3. **Heat Bi:**
   a. DU 14; b. U.B. 11; c. L.I4, d. L.I 11
4. **Vessel Bi: Lu. 9**
5. **Painful Bi.**
   a. K.3　b. L.I 4　c. U.B 11　d. U.B 23
6. **Tendon Bi:**
   a. G.B 34, b. L.I 4, c. Liv 3.

USE OF LOCAL POINTS:

1. Shoulder pain: L.I 15
2. Scapular Pain: U.B. 43
3. Elbow pain: L.I 11
4. Wrist pain: T.W 4
   　　　L.I 5
5. Hip pain: G.B 30
6. Knee pain: U.B. 40
   　　St. 35

7. Ankle pain St. 41
       K.3
8. Lumbar pain: DU 3
9. Stiffness of fingers: Ex.28
    and toes: Ex.36
10. Calf pain: U.B 57
       G.B 34

In addition to these points, Ah. shi points must be selected. Bleeding with cupping is beneficial. In few cases moxibustion is also advisable.

Let us take few arthritic problems in details with the specific point selection.

Name of disease	Points selected.
1. Cervical spondylitis	U.B 10, G.B20 G.B21, U.B11, D u14, Ex 21, S I6, L.I4, Lu7, Tw 5, S.I9.
2. Carpal Tunnel syndrome	Lu9, P6, H7, Sp9, G.B34, L.I 4, Lu10, Du14, U.B11, Ex. 28
3. Frozen shoulder	St 38, G.B34, U.B60, L.I4, L.I15, T.W 14.
4. Tennis elbow	L.I12, L.I 11, L.I10, T.W10, G.B34.
5. Golfer's elbow:	H3, P3, S.I3.
6. Miner's elbow:	T.W10, T.W11, S.I8, L.I4.
7. Pain wrists	S J4, L I5, S.I5, S.J5.
8. Ankylosing spondylitis	U.B11, K.3, U.B. 23, L.I4, Lu7, U.B.40. Ex. 21, Du14, Du11. G.B.30, U.B. 32.
9. Arthritis of hips:	G.B 30, U.B. 37. G.B. 29.
10. Knee pains:	S.t34, St35, Ex.32, G.B34, G.B33, U.B57, U.B 58, Sp9.

Only a brief description is given. The points are selected according to the causative and precipitating factors which are different in every individual case. Similar points are used for acupressure but the technique used is high gravity pressure, small magnets, beads and pellets instead of needles.

HOMOEOPATHIC MANAGEMENT

Homoeopathy as we know is not only a science but an art also. It aims at providing the correct guided stimulus which exists both on the mental, physical and spiritual levels. This system was started by Dr. Christian Bernard Samuel Hahnemann who clearly mentions about the **"Concepts of Similia Similibus Curanter",**

The Law of minimum and single dose.

On the other hand he has equally mentioned about various obstructive factors which have a hindrance and shall obstruct the path of management and cure. According to Dr. Hahnemann in section 3. of organon he has clearly mentioned regarding the removal of cause. In today's modern era the concept of disease and health have changed. So different ways and means have been devised to go for the management. As we know there are different modes of prescription. So let us study them in detail keeping in mind various concepts of disease.

1. **Constitutional prescribing:** It is one of the most difficult means to be adopted in deep seated chronic diseases. It helps us study the miasmatic background and the constitutional analysis of the case. It requires all the necessary details of the patient, his sickness and the person as a whole.

    The constitution can be either carbogenoid hydrogenoid or nitrogenous constitution. Few commonly used remedies in the constitutional group are Calcarea carb, Calcrea phos, Natrum mur, Staphsagria, Nat. sulph., Arsenic alb., etc.

2. **On the basis of L.S.M.C.:** (Location sensation modality

and concomittants. The prescription on the basis of location is not of a much value. But the modalities defenitely help.

Let us look at few examples

Sensation as if

1.	Fatigue were for ever banished	Cann. sat.
2.	Body and limbs did not touch the bed	Sticta.
3.	Glowing in air as if on Brain	Sabadilla
4.	Frail and easily broken	Thuja

ETIOLOGICAL CLASSIFICATION

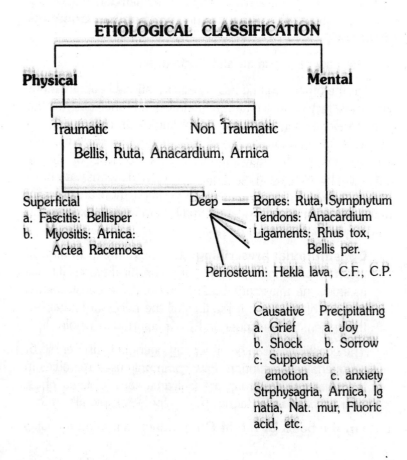

Physical   **Mental**

Traumatic   Non Traumatic

Bellis, Ruta, Anacardium, Arnica

Superficial   Deep —— Bones: Ruta, Symphytum
a. Fascitis: Bellisper   Tendons: Anacardium
b. Myositis: Arnica: Ligaments: Rhus tox,
   Actea Racemosa   Bellis per.

Periosteum: Hekla lava, C.F., C.P.

Causative   Precipitating
a. Grief   a. Joy
b. Shock   b. Sorrow
c. Suppressed
   emotion   c. anxiety
Strphysagria, Arnica, Ig
natia, Nat. mur, Fluoric
acid, etc.

$\rightarrow$

CAUSES/ETIOLOGY

Prodromal Stage $\rightarrow$ **Primary Symptoms**

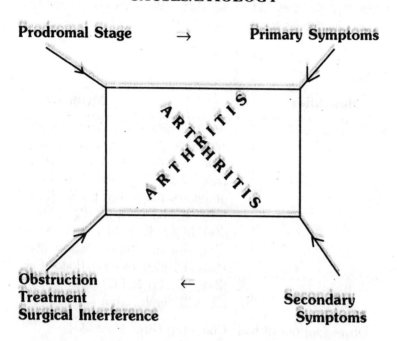

Obstruction $\leftarrow$
Treatment
Surgical Interference   **Secondary**
                                           Symptoms

I. Cure
II . Treatment
III. Management

MODALITIES AND ITS ROLE

To choose a better prescription we can always use modalities as one of the basis of prescription which helps to improve and widen the the scope of prescription. WE have considered few general modalities for reference.

Modalities	Medicine
1. Night << in General	Acon., Agar (2+), Alum., Am-c., Aln., Ars. (2+) Asaf., Aur (2), Bry., Calc., C. veg., Cham. (3+), Cinnb, Dulc., Fers (2+), Flac (2+), Gels., graph., Hep (2+), Kali-bi., K. c(2), K. I. (2), Kalm., Lach (2), Lyc., Merc. (3+), M.J.F. (2+), Merc. sul., Mez., (2+), Nat m., Nit-a., Nux v (2+), Phos., Phyt (2), Plb (3+), Podo., Puls (2+), Rhod (2), R.T (2). Sabin., Sars., (2), S(2), Syph., Thuj.
2. Drives him out of bed	Cham (3), Ferr., Merc (3+)
3. << from cold air	Ars. (3), Daph., Kali-ar., Kalm (2), Sel (2), Tarent (28)
4. << Change of weather	Calc (2), Rhod (3), Sil (2)
5. << coition after	Sil (3), Tub.
6. >> By coffee	Arg-m.
7. << Lying on	Ars. (2), Bry., Iod., Lyc., Merc (2), Nux-v., Rhus t., Verat.
8. Pressure Agg.	Cina., Cocc., Merc., Plb.
9. After Parturition <<	Rhod.

10. Over heated & exertion << Zinc. (2)

11. << In warm weather   Colch (3+) Kali bi (2)

12. Violent exercise <<   Aesculus

13. Warmth of bed agg << Warmth of bed agg << Apis.,
Lac. can (2+), Led (2), Merc. (3),
Phyt., Stel., S (2), Verat (2), Chin.,
Ruta.

14. << Lying down   Chin., Ruta.

15. Pressure amel.   Bry., Form.

16. << During sleep   Sul-ac.

17. Walking, after amel.   Sul-ac.

18. << wine after   Led (2)*

19. << Piano   Led (2+)

20. << Washing with

    cold water   Am-c., Ars.(2)

21. << in winters   Petr.

22. Pain shoulder pressure

    amel.   Coc-c., Nat-c.

23. Putting the arm

    behind him agg.   Ferr (3), Rhus-t. (2), Sanic (3)

For a better evaluation let us divide the groups of medicines into different categories depending on the requirement.

1. **Carbon group:** It includes Carbo vegetabilis and Carbo animalis. When the constitution profile is weak with complaints usually out of control select a Carbon group.

2. **Natrum group:** When there is a repeat history of malarial attacks with a constitutional change specially due to chronic

mental stress, H/o grief etc. It can be Nat. mur., Nat. sulph., Nat. carb. also.

3. **Zincum group:** It usually indicates the involvement of peripheral joints, spine bones with immense weakness. Affecting the nerves thereby accessory symptoms of numbness paraesthesia are noticed with symptoms of arthritis. It usually includes Zincum metallicum, Zincum valeriana and Zincum phosphoricum. It is also suitable to both younger and older age groups.

4. **Plumbum group:** It is indicated when too much morning stiffness is noticed with atrophic changes in the joint. It is also indicated in parkinsons and ankylosing spondylitis. Mental obsessiveness is strongly associated.

5. **Acid Group:** It usually includes: Acetic acid, Nitric acid, Acid carbolic, Acid lacticum etc. It is usually indicated in complicated Arthritis when super added diabetes, hypertension and neurological disturbances are noticed.

6. **Calcarea Group:** It is one of the significant group indicated in arthritis. It includes calcarea carb., Calcarea phos., Calc. lactophos., Calc. hypophos and Calc. ars. It is indicated in cretinism, cushing's syndrome and also in T.B. Arthritis.

7. **Arsenic group:** It includes Arsenic met, Arsenic album., Arsenicum, sul. rubrum, Ars. sulph., Stibiatum when degeneration has set in with evening rise of temperature, emaciation, pallor and extreme debility. It is also indicated in syphilitic arthritis when nocturnal pains at midnight are strongly marked.

8. **Snake poisons:** It includes Lachesis, Crotalus horridus which shows the mixed features of Scleroderma with a haemorrhagic tendency. It is also indicated in varicose veins.

9. **Ammonium salts:** They usually include Ammonium carbonicum, Amm. causticum, Ammonium phos. which helps us in improving general circulation. These patient are quite chubby and fair complexion, chilly but highly sensitive to slightest change of weather.

10. **Baryta group:** It includes Baryta carb., Baryta iod, Baryta mur. It is also applicable when arthritic complications are associated with cardiovascular symptoms.

11. **Kali group:** It usually has all the polycrests which are highly beneficial when oedema and or Ascrites is predominately associated with marked anaemia. Clubbing and respiratory distress also.

12. **Magnesia group:** It includes Magnesia carb., Mag. sulph., Mag. mur., when it has magnesium with iron which helps in Reiter's disease, enteropathic gastritis etc.

13. **Bowel nosodes:** They include proteus bach, baccilus No. 7., Sycotic co., Morgan Gartener.

14. **Nosodes and Sarcodes:** They are used both as intercurrent and initiating remedies they include Medorrhinum, Psorinum, Pyrogenium, Tuberculinum, Bacillinum etc.

15. **Glandular Remedies:** They include corpus leuteum, Parathyroid, Pituitary, X-ray, Thyroidinum, Mammary, Pineal. They all are available in either 3x or 6x potency.

16. A list of rare Remedies:

    1. Apocyanum Androsemifolium

    2. Sterculia: In low dilutions or mother tincture.

    3. Methylene blue in 3x trituration

    4. Stellaria media: In mother tincture

    5. Indigo

    6. Ilex cassine

    7. Iridium

    8. Gettysburg water.

    9. Homarus

    10. Momordica

    11. Upas Tienta

12. Apomorphine

13. Scirrhinum.

14. Scrophularia nodosa.

15. Paris quadrifolia.

16. Lonicella.

17. Thallium met.

18. Thevita.

19. T.N.T.

20. Taxus bacata.

21. Sol.

22. Luna.

23. Magnets polus arctiicus.

24. Magnetis poli ambo.

25. Magnolia glauca.

Let us take up few rare and uncommon but useful drugs.

The selection of medicines becomes quite easy when it is in groups. It helps to improve and search our knowledge rather than depending on the ready made feast. We aim at individualisation so select your own remedy.

LET US TAKE UP FEW RARE AND UN-
COMMON BUT USEFUL DRUGS

1. **Itchyol:** It has a strong antiseptic and antiinflammatory properties. It is highly beneficial in gout and rheumatoid arthritis. It has been used only on the symptom of acute pains.

2. **Ictodes:** It is skunk weed which found in California. It is useful in rheumatoid arthritis with burning palms and soles as a predominant symptom.

3. **Illicium anisatum:** The star-anise belongs to magnoliaceae. It is useful in ankylosing spondylitis and acute lumbar spondylitis. It is also used in intercostal neuralgia and post herpetic neuralgia.

4. **Indigo:** It is a mixed oxidation product of several plant juices mainly Indigofera tinctoria. It is useful in Lumbo sciatica syndrome when the specific nocturnal aggravation at 3 a.m. > by moving and pressure.

5. **Indium:** It derieves it's name from the blue spectrum of indigo blue. It has some similarities to titanium and selenium. It is also useful in **Lumbar spondylosis** with radiating pains felt only in soles of feet. It is useful in frozen shoulder, cervical spondylitis and extra rib syndrome.

6. **Inula:** It is a perennial plant which is used primarily in Lumbo sciatica syndrome when the pain is associated with **Genito urinary symptoms,** affecting the (R) side. It is also useful in neuralgia pains of **A Vascular Necrosis (A.V.N.)**

7. **iodoformum:** It is useful in Koch's Arthritis specially affecting the knee joints and the spine. Pains << slightest efforts to stand with radiation down both antero lateral aspects of thighs.

8. **Iridium:** It is a heavy metal of Platinum group. Pains with numbness is the primary symptom left sided sciatica preventing sleep. Pain in both knees << bending but > by pressing upper thighs.

9. **Iris versi color:** This blue flag is a known remedy for non insulin dependent diabetes but recommended in psoriatic arthritis with burning tips of fingers. All the complaints are agg at night and by movement.

10. **ITU:** It is an alcoholic solution of resin. It is a useful remedy in cervical spasm when stiffness is well marked.

11. **Jacaranda caroba:** It has a palliative role in syphilitic arthropathy and helps in Gonorrhoeal rheumatism. It is useful in cervical spondylosis when neck movement "leading to nausea:

12. **Jasminum:** It is the famous jasmine and is useful in non specific arthritis when tiredness is out of proportion.

13. **Jatropha:** The physic nut belongs to euphorbiaceace and is indicated in calcanean spurs. When sharp pricking pains are marked.

15. **Jequirity:** The Indian liquorice belongs to leguminosae and is indicated in Charcoat's joints when painlessness is predominant.

15. **Juglans cinerea:** It is useful in scleroderma and radiating pains of neuropathy when slightest walking << the pains.

16. **Juncus:** It is indicated in generalised nonspecific arthralgia when lower back is affected. Pains are always associated with rectal tenesmus. Therefore it is useful in intestinal arthropathy of auto immune origin.

17. **Kali chloricum:** It is the chlorate of potassium which is indicated in rheumatoid arthritis and also in syphilitic arthritis when extreme debility, morning pains and associated gastric symptoms are reknowned.

18. **Kali cyanatum:** It is useful in Rheumatoid arthritis, S.L.E. when 2nd advanced stage with destruction and cyanosis of extremities is marked.

19. **Kali iodide:** This is Kali hydroidium which is indicated in T.B. arthritis, non specific arthritis when only ESR is moderately raised. It is useful in baker's cyst, housemaid's knee, bursitis, rheumatoid arthritis when affecting the knee joints in secondary stage.

20. **Kali Nitricum:** It is indicated in arthritis of syphilitic origin when pains are worse at night with slightest aggravation from draft of air, < by coffee >> by lying on right side and uncovering head.

21. **Kali oxalicum:** Oxalate of potassium is useful in syphilitic arthritis with increased frequency of urination.

22. **Kaolin:** The China clay is useful in intercostal neuralgia and non specific arthritis. It is usually associated with croupous laryngitis.

23. **Karaka:** It is useful in arthritis affecting the ankles only with fibrositis affecting the soles of feet.

24. **Kissingen:** It is a compound water with sodium chloride as one of the leading compounds. Painful, cramps legs with arthritic pains affecting knees and ankles. Pains << damp weather.

25. **Laburnum:** It belongs to leguminosae and the mother tincture is prepared from the fresh bark. It is indicated in the vascular compression symptoms due to cervical spondylosis which is postural vertigo with dizziness. Dizziness is always associated with twitching of muscles.

26. **Lachnanthes:** L. Tinctoria, the red root is useful in spasmodic torticolis or wry neck specially affecting the right side of neck. Constant sensation as if nostrils are pinched together.

27. **Lacticum acidicum:** The sour milk was 1st discovered by

Scheele under the influence of casein. It is usually indicated in diabetic neuropathy, rheumatoid arthritis affecting both knees with increased salivation. It is useful in sciatica affecting the right side. **All pains are better by eating.**

28. **Lathyrus:** Check pea belongs to leguminosae and the mother tincture is prepared from the seeds. It is useful in lumbago, << lying ddown > by raising the legs. It is indicated in calcanean spur and plantar fascitis.

29. **Lepidium bunariense:** It is the brazillian cress, very commonly found along the roads and in stony regions of mure. It is indicated in nonspecific arthritis when excruciating pains are very marked.

30. **Oxytropis lamerti:** "Luco seed" is useful in osteoarthrosis when pain is << thinking of it, << immediately after eating and > in cool air.

31. **Pediculus:** It is useful in psoriatic arthritis when pains are associated with formication.

32. **Rhus venenata:** It is one of the most active poisonous of Rhus. It is indicated in lumbago, lumbo sciatica affecting right side. Pains as if skin is scalded.

33. **Rubia tinctoria:** It is specially indicated in syphillitic affections of bones, lordosis and plantar fascitis.

34. **Saccharum lactis:** It is one of the inert group of medicines founded by Hahnemann it is indicated primarily in gout, rheumatoid arthritis affection knees, pains > lying on left side **<< from sound of running water.**

35. **Silica marina:** It is prepared from the sea beach and is useful in gonorrhoeal rheumatism and syphilitic arthritis affecting primarily the knee joints.

36. **Slag:** It is the melt of iron sillico sulphate prepared from the furnace. It is used in a bursitis, capsulitis, housemaid's knee. **Creeping chill is always associated with pains.**

37. **Stachys betonica:** It is useful in dizziness of cervical spondylosis << standing only.

38. **Stellaria media:** Initially it was used locally on the inflammed joints. It is now used internally in acute pains as if string were pulled from ear to shoulder. Darting pains in shoulder blade with radiation upto the neck. Indicated in cervical spondylosis with radiating neuralgic pains on left side.

39. **Linum catharaticum:** It is a purging plant and the mother tincture is prepared from the whole plant. It is indicated in cervical and lumbar spondylosis with radiating neuralgic pains.

40. **Lithium Benzoicum:** It is useful in gout and gouty arthritis when increased urinary frequency is the main associated complaint.

41. **Lithium lacticum:** It affects primarily the shoulders subacute capsulitis and radiating cervical neuropathy. It is highly beneficial in rheumatoid arthritis when it affects the elbows and shoulders only.

42. **Napthalinum:** It is the distillation product of coal tar containing colorless, transparent scales. It is useful in psoriatic arthritis.

43. **Natrum lacticum:** It is useful in gout and arthritis when unusual hunger and thirst is associated with them.

44. **Nuphar leuteum:** It is indicated in psoratatic and gouty arthritis when associated with diarrhoea as one of the concomitant symptom, aggravation between 4-6 a.m.

45. **Oleum jecoris Aselli:** The cod liver oil is obtained from the liver of gadus morrhua and some other fish. It is used in right sided sciatica, lumbago pains > by pressure. It is used in rheumatoid arthritis when pains are very strongly marked.

46. **Ostrya:** It is indicated in osteoarthritis when repeat attacks of malaria are associated as in gouty arthritis, rheumatoid

of knees when pains << slightest efforts from << Darting pains small joints of middle and index fingers of one hand only.

47. **Stillingia sylvatica:** It is a popular remedy in syphilitic arthritis, in Reiter's disease, rheumatoid arthritis affecting the knees and metatarsus pains << slightest exposure to air aggravate.

48. **Strontium carb:** It is indicated in rheumatoid arthritis affecting ankles only. Pain in tendons as if stretched << exertion, movement, > by movement of right arm.

49. **Tanacetum:** It is useful in syphilitic arthritis when bony protrusions are well marked with severe darting pains << slightest touch, air contact of.

50. **Tanin:** It is useful in autoimmune compound presentations **when diarrhoea is always an associated symptom.**

51. **Taxus bacata:** Mother tincture is prepared from the young shoots. It is indicated in gout, rheumatoid arthritis when pains are << by pressure, < application of liquids.

SURGICAL MANAGEMENT

The role of surgery begins when the scope of physical medicine ends. We have heard very bright stories about surgical intervention but we must know what to do and when. Surgery is successful when all the possible modes have been failed.

An expert opinion is given for surgery only when all other resources have been exhausted. Since 1960's with the beginning of surgical orthopaedics a new light has been given to the totally disabled or even crippled cases. But we must know the facts regarding the surgery also.

Indications of surgery:

1. Complete failure to restore the normal activities.

2. Multiple arthritis with immediate need for rehabilitation.

3. Intra-articular damages not being under the scope of physical means or medicines.

Hindrances in surgery:

1. Diabetes and hypertension.

2. Obesity with secondary complications.

3. Any chronic infection interfering with the general resistance of body.

TERMINOLOGY IN THE SURGERY:

1. **Arthrodesis:** It is also known as bone fusion. It is done mainly in ankles and wrists to relieve pain. When they are fused or frozen, they are not flexible but without pain.

2. **Arthroplasty:** Restructuring the joint is called arthroplasty. It involves resurfacing or relining the ends of bones where the cartilage has worn away and destruction of bone has occurred. It is also known as prosthesis of joint.

3. **Arthroscopy:** It aims at visualising the inner of joints by looking through a thin instrument called an arthroscope. It is inserted through a 6 mm incision. It is done under local anaesthesia.

4. **Arthrotomy:** During this procedure the joints are surgically opened to allow accurate diagnosis and make surgical repairs.

5. **Osteotomy:** It is done to correct bone deformities or improper allignment of the bone. The surgeon cuts and resets the bone, allowing it to heal in a better position.

6. **Resection:** Removal of a bone or pat of the bone is called bone resection. It is used in painful bunions and in metatarsals of feet.

7. **Synovectomy:** It aims at opening of joint and removing the membrane inflamed by arthritis.

SURGICAL TECHNIQUES

Hip joint: Two types of techniques are used. One is total hip replacement and the other is resurfacing. The choice of procedure depends on the need of patient resurfacing involves cleaning away the top of thigh bone and lapping it with a metal covering. Hip joint socket is cleaned and lined with a plastic material.

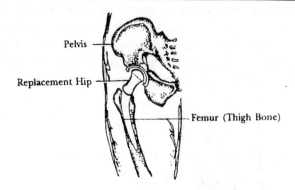

Total Hip Joint Replacement

Knee joint: The major procedure is arthroscopy followed by total or partial joint replacement. It helps in overcoming severe distress to the joint.

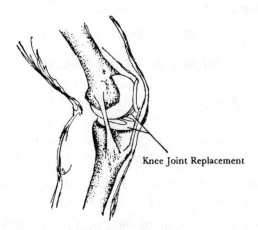

Knee Replacement

Elbow joint: Synovectomy is accompanied by resection. But it is not very useful.

Shoulder: Pain can occasionally be helped by arthroscopy. In few cases total joint replacement helps.

Ankle and foot: Arthrodesis is commonly done in foot. When the metatarsal arch is painful, resection of heads is advised.

Hands and wrists: Tenosynovectomy is done to relieve the distressing pain of tenosynovitis. Sometimes a tendon repair is also needed, to correct the deformity in crippling hand and foot deformity Silicon rubber implants are used. Arthrodesis helps in relieving the pains.

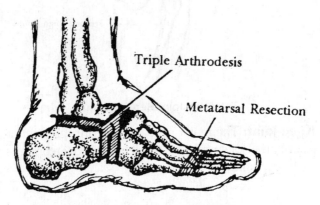

Sites of Two Types of Foot Surgery

Limitations after Surgery

1. It may not be necessary to revive the same old gait or walking capacity.

2. For the maintenance physical means have to be continued which helps in the long run.

3. Sometimes post surgical complications may be seen which should be taken care of.

4. Some limitations of movements may remain after surgery.

Therefore after understanding each aspect we must conclude that even surgery is useful if indicated.

Clinical Case Records

Patient's Record	Clinical Symptoms & Diagnosis	Treatment Given
1. Mrs. Anju Sondhi 28/F	- Limping while walking - Numbness (L) Leg - 1yr. Δed: with investigations L_4-L_5 Sacrilization	Homoeopathic Medicine Argentum Nitricum 10M few doses - Lumbar Traction 20 Kgx15 min. & Ultrasonic radiations x 10 days. - Response good. Now only on maintenance homoeopathic treatment.
2. Mr. Sanjeev Sondhi 33/M	- Numbness both legs with easy tiredness. - 1½ year - Gastric upset Δed: L_4-L_5 mild disc prolapse	Homoeopathic Medicine - Medorrhinum 10M 3 doses. - TENS for 20 min. - Lumbar traction 30 Kg x 10 days Follow up good gradually physiotherapy withdrawn.Response, good, now on maintenence treatment.
3. Mr. Amarjeet Singh 38/M.	- Pain Radiation down both legs - Pain lumbar & sacral region - 3 yrs. Δed disc prolapse Δed disc prolapse	Sepia 1M followed by rubmet for 2-3 wks. with follow up of hydrofluoric acid.

4. Mr. Lalit Thapar. 29/M	- Pain severe neck and upper dorsum back - 10/15 days Δed: X-ray C.spine, ESR & Calcium levels.	- Acupuncture at K.3, Du14, U.B60, U.B54. - Response good, now on homoeopathic and Acupuncture follow up. Started with Rhus tox 1M. Physiotherapy - Cervical traction 10 Kg x 12 min. - S.W.D. x 10 min. for 10 days. Still being followed up. Now >>
5. Mrs. Kanta Govil 56/F	- Poly rheumatoid arthritis with hypertention - 15/16 yrs. - Spindle joint deformities - 3rd stage arthritis but could maintain herself.	Started with various homoeopathic medicines - Initially with ultrasonic - No relief. - Acupuncture initially mild response but gradually no response. Case needed surgical management.
6. Mrs. Urmil Kapoor 42/F	- Pain (L) knee joint: - 16 months - Had an accident with fracture upper end of fibula advised bed rest for 3 months. - After recovery developed arthritic changes of secondary with stiffness, inability to move and pain on continuous walking	Started Hepar sulph. Followed by Kali sulph., Medorrhinum and Argent. but the case settled down with Lycopodium. - Acupuncture at K_3, St_{36}, $G.B_{34}$ with Sujok combination. Good response now on both acupuncture and homoeopathic management

7.	Mrs. Deepa Chhabra 32/F	Had an episode of throat viral suspected which was followed by sudden onset of severe crippling pains leading to complete immobility - 10 days Δed rheumatic fever by raised ASO titre, Raised E.S.R. Echocardiography showed few desposits. E.S.R. evaluated W.N.L.	Homoeopathic medicines, included, Kali bich (Q), Scirrhinum, Syphillinum, accordingly. - Given 6-7 sittings of TENS. - Acupuncture both classical and Sujok. Non completely taken care of totally mobile. Now without acupuncture sittings but only on Homoeopathic management.
8.	Mrs. Kailash Gupta 55/F	- Pain (R) shoulder with mild radiation to neck Δed Capsulitis with frozen shoulder - 1 month	Started initially with homoeopathic medicines • Tens and ultrasonic x 15 days. It gave her only mild relief. - It was followed by acupuncture for nearly 20-30 sittings which made her recover almost 75-80-%. But she could not continue the treatment further. Is on homoeopathic management only for pain relief.
9.	Mrs. Nirmal Sibbal 60/F	A chronic rheumatoid arthritis with crippling deformities - 20 yrs. but	

10. Sunil Chhabra 35/M	2 years back completely immobile - Stiffness I.P. joints - 1 month - Δed early R.A. with raised E.S.R. positive RA factor E.S.R. evaluatedafter treatment came to normal levels.	Acupuncture helps her to cover stiffness and few secondary symptoms. - Adv. surgical management with knee joint replacement. Advised wax (paraffin) for 10 days. Medorrhinum in homoeopathic management response - good. Only ocassional Pain << change of weather. Now no treatment.
11. Mr. Sudhir Thukral 46/M	- Pain knee joints - 2 yrs. - Pain ankles - 2 yrs. - Pain lower back - 4/5 yrs. Δed hyperurecemia with ankylosing spondylitis (HLAB27 +ve) with MRI findings confirmed	Is on homoeopathic management in between few sittings of S.W.D./Lumbar traction and I.F.T. were given. It is followed by nature cure and homoeopathic management.
12. Mrs, Bhupinder Kaur 40/F	- Pain both knees - 2 yrs. Δed early osteoarthritic changes	Patient had already been on nature cure for a year. Now she is under purely homoeopathic

13. Mrs. Jaggi 58/F	- Pain both knees: 8/9 yrs. Δed Osteoarthrosis both knee joints (3rd stage)	management. Nat. mur was the constitutional prescription. Started homoeopathic medication. X-ray 1M with X-ray in low potency. It was associated with acupuncture but she could be given nearly 60% relief. She is now only on medication.
14. Mrs. Saroj Gupta 46/F	Rheumatoid arthritis with osteo-arthritis both knee joints - 10 yrs. ESR moderately increased with osteoporotic changes.	Started with homoeopathic management and acupuncture she is maintaining a pain free period.
15. Mrs. Seeta Rao 62/F	Δed T.B. Arthritis. - 5/6 yrs. Both knee joints ESR 95 mm/1st hour Mantoux: 30/20 mm 1st reading. After nearly six months Mantox 10/15 mm and ESR 55mm/1st hr. Now ESR between 40-50 mm/1st hr.	Started with acupuncture & homoeopathic management. She is comfortable but still has lot of postural problems.

17. Mr. Narender Bhanot 49/M	C/o numbness both feet and heaviness legs. Δed coppmression at L_4-L_5 S_1	Given acupuncture only. Follow up awaited.
18. Miss Rani Jagpal 22/F	- Pain (L) elbow Δed T.B. bursitis	Given ultrasonic radiations. No response - Acupuncture no response she did not come for further follow up.
19. Miss Anjali Varma 22/F	- Pain neck with radiation down (R) arm MRI shows only cervical spasm.	Came to the centre after taking ultrasonic I.F.T. but no relief. started acupuncture. Now much comfortable with both acupuncture and medicine (c-c 10M) was the constitutional remedy.
20. Mrs.Sunita Aggarwal 60/F	- Chronic rheumatoid arthritis with osteo arthrosis both knees - 30 yrs.	Given all complimentary treatments of Physiotherapy, acupuncture. But did not respond to any of the therapies. Advised general management.
21.Mrs. Neetu Aggarwal 22/F	- Pain lumbosacral region Δed sacro ileitis.	Moschus was the constitutional remedy.

22. Mrs. Ved Sharma 59/F	- Dizziness with headache, pain neck and back Δed cervical spondylosis with lumbar spondylosis	- Cervical and lumbar traction with ultrasonic x 10 days.
23. Mrs. Bimla 50/F	- Numbness with paresthesiae both hands/feet - 1 year. - Borderline diabetic Δed cervical myelopathy	- Acupuncture in few sittings did not give her benefit. She did not report back for follow up.
24. Mrs. Neera Mohini Nigam 58/F	- Pain both knees - 3 months Δed O.A. both knees	Is on homoeopathic management
25. Mrs. Sujata 33/F	- Pain both knees; elbows - 3/4 years. Δed rheumatoid arthritis with raised E.S.E./RA factor +ve.	Is on homoeopathic management. In between 2-3 cources of acupuncture and ultrasonic radiations are given. She is under a maintenance regmen.
26. Mr. S.V. Shende 55/M	- Pain both knees: 10/15 days Δed O.A. (early)	Gave only 10 sittings of acupuncture - Good response. Now symptom free.

Patient	Clinical	Management
27. Mrs. Manjula Shende 52/F	- Pain (R) shoulder with restricted movements - 3 months	Given only TENS and ultrasonic for x 20 days. Response - +ve.
28/Mr. P.C. Arora 63/M	- Dizziness << lying on (L) or on back straight. CT Scan shows disc compression at C_5-C_6	Given only acupuncture of 10-12 sittings. Response - Good. Now on Homoeopathic management only.
30. Mrs. Ruby Kharbanda 29 /F	- Pain back with Radiation down (R) Leg/thigh Δed L_4L_5 Sacralization	Given Tens and Ultrasonic for follow up.
31. Mrs. Pushpa Sachdeva 60/F	Chronic osteoarthrosis both knee joints - 10 yrs. 3rd stage with complete destruction of cartilage	Started with homoeopathic medicines. In between acupuncture and physiotherapy were given with a minimal relief. She is on homoeopathic maintenance.
32. Mr. Raju 32/M	- Pain neck with heavines. 3/4 months. Δed cervical spasm	Cervical traction and neck exercises restored completely.

33. Mr.J.L. Tikku 56/M	- Pain neck with occasional dizziness. Δed cervical spondylosis	Given cervical traction for few days response - Good
34. Mohd. Haquvi 42/M	Pain neck with loss of neck movements - 10 yrs. Δed Ankylosing spondylitis with HLAB$_{27}$ +ve and raised ESR.	Started with acupuncture. But the patent did not pursue to continue the treatment.
35. Harmohinder Bajaj 60/F	Chronic arthritis with non-specific complications - 10/11 yrs.	Mainly on homoeoapthic management (Thyroidinum) was the drug of choice.
36. Mrs. Mithlesh Mathur 62/F	Chronic painful joints generalised 10/yrs.	Only on homoeoapthic management.
37. Mrs. Krishna Batra 68/F	Chronic O.A. knees with obesity of 2nd grade	Initially given acupuncture. But she did not pursue the treatment.
38. Bhagya Shree 20/F	Presented with chronic arthritic pains. 24 yrs. Δed as early rheumatoid arthritis	Only on homoeoapthic management.

9. Mrs. Sudesh Bhaskar 50/F	- Pain (L) elbow Δed as tennis elbow.	Ultrasonic radiations helped her.
10. Mr. Y.P. Chaudhary 68/M	- Burning and pain soles of feet 2 yrs. Occasional pain lower back - 1 yr. Δed: L_4-L_5 disc prolapse	Started with TENS and ultrasonic. Recovery good.
11. Mrs. Narottam Khosla 44/F	- Pain (R) shoulder Δed frozen shoulder with acute cervical spondylosis	Only on homoeopathic management. Lac. def. was the remedy.
42. Mrs. Sheela Rana 40 /F	Chronic Rheumatoid Arthritis. Affecting nearly all joints-5/6 yrs.	Only on homoeopathic management. Scirrhinum 1M with Methyl blue helped.
43. Mr. Dinesh Bansal 35/M	- Pain both calf muscles with muscles contractions. Δed varicose veins	Only on Homoeopathic management. Acid nit. in Q. helped him.
44. Mrs. Kailash Sondhi 65/F	Chronic Polyarthritis with predominant osteolytic deposits	Given acupuncture with failure Homoeopathic management but the patients did not pursue further.

Name	Symptoms	Notes
45. Mrs. Renu Tikku	- Dizziness with occasional pains, back	Only 5-6 sitting of nedles made her comfortable.
46. Mrs. Shail Narang 33/F	- Chronic generalised bodyaches since long. Δed bordering hypothyroidism	Only on homoeopathic medication but her obesity programming is also conducted.
47. Mrs. Shanta Sharma 60/F	- Chronic numbness feet with inability to walk to raise a step Δed neuropathy	Acupuncture helped her slightly. Now on medicine only. (Silicea)
48. Mr. Omprakash 44/M	- Pain both knee joint - 2 yrs. Δed osteoarthritis with the help of ESR. and X-ray knees.	Given only Acupuncture. He gives a good response. But the treatment could not be completed.
49. Mr. D.K. Sud 50/M	- Pain multiple joints Δed rheumatoid arthritis	Is on homoeopathic management. Medorrhinum 10 M/3 doses
50. Mrs. Janjna Devi 75/F	- Pain both ankles, knees-3/4 yrs. - Numbness soles of feet Δed peripheral neuropathy with O.A. knees.	Is only on homoeopathic management. She moves with restricted activities.

51. Mrs. Santosh Jain 33/F	- Pain lower back with radiation to (R) leg.	Given only physiotherapy ultrasonic, TENS for few days made her comfortable.
52. Mr. Sanjay Tikku	- Pain (L) ankle - 10 days Date back to sprain Δed fibrositis ankle with capsulitis	Given wax paraffin x 10 days. Followed by ultrasonic x 15 days Resported to be O.K.
53. Mrs. Pushpa Sehgal 58/F	- Pain both knees 5/6 yrs.	Adv: Wax treatment along with homoeopathic management. Comfortable.
54. Mrs. Renu Miglani 40/F	- Pain lumbar region had exertion Δed L_4–L_5 disc prolapse With chipped fracture L_4 vertebrae	Adv.: Lumbar cast, TENS and wax x 10 days. Reported better.
55. Mrs. Usha Gupta 42/F	- Pain (R) shoulder - 10/15 days Δed frozen shoulder	- Acupuncture - X 10 days. - Ultrasonic and tens did not give her a complete relief.
56. Mrs. Shashi Kapoor 55/F	- Chronic arthralgic pains both knees - 10 yrs.	On homoeoapthic management with few sittings of acupuncture were given.
57. Mrs. Randhava 82/F	- Pain both ankles Δed osteoporotic bone changes	Ultrasonic on ankles x 10 days. Pain and swelling relieved.

58. Mr. S.K. Grover 60/M	- Pains both causes and occasionally on back Δed peripheral neuritis	Acupuncture only U.B$_{60}$, K$_3$, G.B$_4$, U.B$_{57}$, Felt > but no follow up.
59. Mrs. Neeti Aggarwal 36/F	- Pain lower back with shifting and radiating pains across abdomen. Δed Lumbar spondylo listhesis	- Physiotherapy and acupuncture along with magnet therapy is given. No apparent change.
60. Mrs. Meena Kothari 63/F	- Chronic lumbago with cervical pains Δed L.S.S. with chronic myelopathy	Is on homoeopathic management. Now Acupuncture is started which helped her tremendously.

The Basic aim of providing different cases is to throw light on different arthritic cases, their presentation so that we can understand the limitations and scope of every system and should guide our patients accordingly I did not feel essential to mention the homoeopathic remedies as the remedy selection is quite controversial and is affected by many factors specifically when each case is to be individualised.

SUMMARISATION TO TAKE UP AND FOLLOW ARTHRITIS

We have already discussed each and every practical aspect of an arthritic case starting from the diagnosis to management and treatment. But there are certain aspects to be emphasised upon. Let us have a brief look upon them

The work of the physician starts from the very first enterance of the patient into his chamber.

1. **Observation and history taking:** Although observation is a part of history taking but in special reference includes the physical aspect of constitution, the presentation so that categorically the patient can be classed into either normosthenic, hypersthenic or hyposhenic constitution profile or into hydrogenoid, carbo nitrogenoid or oxygenoid constitution colors.

2. **Clinical and morphological examination:** It includes specific examination of orthopaedic system which includes the gait, physiological deformities, scoliosis, lordosis, duptyren's contracture, osler's nodes, hebreden's nodes, muscle wasting etc.

3. **Studying and analysing the case both according to:** The pathology and the type of adopted treatment. It helps to diagnose the case and manage it accordingly whether it falls in 1st, 2nd or 3rd stage and what all complementary modes of treatment are to be adopted (already discussed)

4. **Management profile:** All the details being discussed.

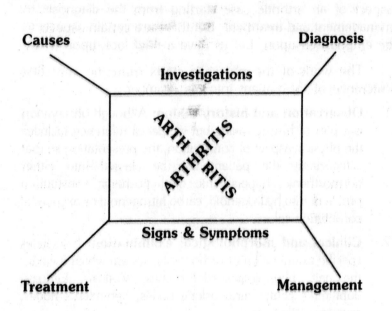

Homoeopathy

- Similia Similibus Curantur
- Law of simple.
  single & minimum

Acupuncture

- Needles
- Electrostimulation
- Moxibustion
- Cupping

ARTHRITIS

Physiotherapy

- Paraffin Wax
- Ultrasonic
- T.E.N.S.
- S.W.D.
- I.F.T.

Nature Cure & Magnetotherapy

- Law of Equalia
- Nature's Law
- Food Cure

SCHEME OF MANAGEMENT OF DISEASE

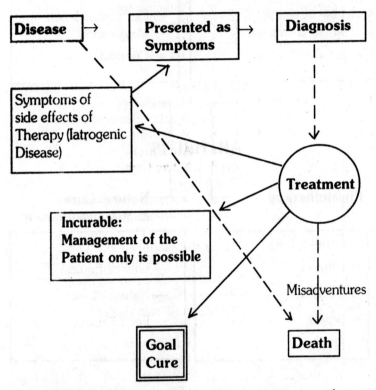

About 35% of patients get beter or have amelioration of symptoms, wherever the therapy administeed. This is known as the **Placebo effect.**

Let us have an analysed look on the therapeutic kits available with us regarding arthritis

Type of Arthritis	Best mode of treatment applicable.

1. Rheumatoid Arthritis

Early Stage
   a. Medicinal Management
   b. Physiotherapy
1. Wax Paraffin
2. S.W.D.
   c. Diet and Regimen
   d. Magnet therapy

2nd Stage
   a. Physiotherapy
      (S.W.D.,Ultrasonic, I.F.T.)
   b. Medicinal management
   c. Acupuncture
   d. Nature Cure

3rd Stage
   a. Medicinal Management ⎤
   b. Acupuncture   ⎥ Only
   c. Surgical Intervention ⎦ Palliative

2. Rheumatic Arthritis

Medicinal Management
Surgical Intervention if only some Cardiac complications are developed.

3. Osteoarthritis

Primary Stage
1. Medicinal Management
2. Physiotherapy
   a. Paraffin wax
   b. Ultrasonic
   c. S.W.D.
   d. I.F.T.
3. Magnet Therapy

Secondary Stage
   a. Medicinal Management
   b. Acupuncture   ⎤ Only paliative &
   c. I.F.T.   ⎥ managing the
             ⎥ cases
Tertiary Stage   ⎦

4. Ankylosing
   spondylitis

    a. Surgical Intervention
   Primary Stage. Mostly it is undiagnosed
   in the primary stage. Therefore only
   medicinal management is given.
   Secondary & Tertiary stage
   a. Acupuncture
   b. Medicinal Management
   To relieve pain only. The fibrosis taken
   place cannot be reversed.

5. Gonococcal arthritis
6. T.B. Arthritis

    Medicinal management
   Medicinal Management (A.T.T.) other
   therapeutic kits can be used to relieve
   pain.

7. Cervical spondylosis
   & Lumbar spondylosis

    1. Primary stage
       a. Physiotherapy and exercises.
       b. Medicinal management.
       c. Magnet therapy.
   2. Secondary Stage
       a. Physiotherapy (I.F.T., Ultrasonic)
       b. Medicine
       c. Acupuncture.
   3. Tertiary stage
       a. Acupuncture
       b. Paliative medicinal management.

It is very important to understand and guide the patient psycology. It can be done by counselling which includes both the solitary and professional counselling also.

They are clinically viewed cases. The individualisation of each and every case is highly important to guide a patient.

In the end we have summarised arthritis in the best possible details with regard to it's etiology, classification, management and treatment. We have understood the applicability of different methods of treatment with their limitations and scope. Let us all make combined efforts towards the achievement of our goal.

Word Index